In My Room

The Author

Professor James V. Lucey MD (Dub), PhD (Lond), FRCPI, FRCPsych is Medical Director, St Patrick's Mental Health Services, Dublin and Clinical Professor of Psychiatry, Trinity College Dublin. He has more than 25 years' experience in psychiatry. In addition to medical management he maintains his clinical practice at St Patrick's where he works on the assessment, diagnosis and management of obsessive compulsive (OCD) and other anxiety disorders. He gives public lectures and is a regular broadcaster on mental health matters on RTÉ Radio, featuring on 'Today with Sean O'Rourke'.

In My Room

The recovery journey as encountered by a psychiatrist

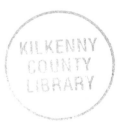
Jim Lucey

Gill & Macmillan

Gill & Macmillan
Hume Avenue, Park West, Dublin 12
www.gillmacmillanbooks.ie

© Jim Lucey 2014
978 07171 5951 2

Typography design by Make Communication
Print origination by O'K Graphic Design, Dublin
Printed and bound by CPI Group (UK) Ltd, Croydon, CR0 4YY

This book is typeset in 11/15 pt Minion

The paper used in this book comes from the wood pulp of managed forests.
For every tree felled, at least one tree is planted, thereby renewing natural
resources.

A CIP catalogue record for this book is available from the
British Library.

5 4 3 2 1

For permission to reproduce copyright material, grateful acknowledgement is
made to the following:

'The Mower' by Philip Larkin from *Philip Larkin Collected Poems*, and 'Post-
script' by Seamus Heaney from *The Spirit Level* by Seamus Heaney, are
reproduced by kind permission of Faber & Faber Ltd.

'The Lost Son,' copyright © 1947 by Theodore Roethke; from *Collected
Poems* by Theodore Roethke. Used by permission of Doubleday, an imprint of
the Knopf Doubleday Publishing Group, a division of Random House LLC. All
rights reserved.

The publishers have made every effort to trace and correctly acknowledge the
copyright holders. If, however, they have inadvertently overlooked any, they
will be pleased to make the necessary arrangements at the first opportunity.

For Philippine

A lively understandable spirit
Once entertained you.
It will come again.
Be still.
Wait.

THEODORE ROETHKE

Contents

Acknowledgements

This book arose from a series of broadcasts on RTÉ Radio about mental health, given between 2009 and 2013. I wish to thank Pat Kenny, Sean O'Rourke and Kay Sheehy, presenters and producer, for inviting me to contribute. Some of this text was previously presented at a lecture in 2009 given in the Abbey Theatre in Dublin prior to a production of a play by Sebastian Barry entitled *Tales of Ballycumber*.

Through the years, I have been fortunate in my teachers and supervisors and my debt to them is very great. I owe a special debt of gratitude to the late Professor Anthony W. Clare, who first encouraged me to write a popular book on therapy for mental disorders when I was his Norman Moore Research Fellow at St Patrick's University Hospital in Dublin.

More recently many friends and colleagues have supported me as I have written drafts of this work. I could not have completed it without their assistance and so I am indebted in a special way to them. They include Sheila Crowley, John Hillery, John O'Mahony, James Braddock, Sarah Surgenor, Anne Donnelly, James Colleran, Charlotte and David Shore, Aidan Halligan, Conor Killeen, Peter Morrogh, Liam Hennessy, Valerie Seymour, Niamh Clarke, David Curtis, Paul Gilligan, Tom Maher, Charlotte Frorath, Kevin Lynch, Seamus Brett and particularly my nephew Eddie Neale.

My special thanks go to my colleague Padraig Wright who is co-editor (along with his colleagues Julian Stern and Michael Phelan) of the authoritative text *Core Psychiatry*, published by Saunders Elsevier and now in its third edition. This is a reference I use regularly in my undergraduate and postgraduate teaching at

St Patrick's University Hospital and at Trinity College Dublin. Many of the ideas I touch upon briefly in this book are elaborated in a more scholarly fashion in the chapters of *Core Psychiatry*.

My thanks go also to Nicki Howard of Gill & Macmillan, and Emma Farrell and Ronan Vaughan of Dog's-ear, who have from the beginning been sources of sustaining enthusiasm.

Lastly, I am very grateful to my wife and family for their love and support.

Author's Note

The author's earnings from sales of this book will be given to the St Patrick's Hospital Foundation in support of the Walk in My Shoes campaign that is raising funds for services for young people with mental health difficulties in Ireland.

Introduction

This book goes some way towards describing my clinical practice. I have done this in the hope that it might demystify the hidden zone that exists between the psychiatrist and the patient, and illuminate in part the journey some people take to mental health and recovery. I have chosen the method of clinical storytelling. Wherever I have included an account it is intended to illustrate a human issue that is derived from a real professional experience. This is not a representative textbook of psychiatry or a manual for self-help, neither is it a comprehensive description of mental health care in Ireland.[1] It is intended for the general reader, as an authentic description of the journey from distress to recovery as I have witnessed it.

My understanding of recovery has grown over many years and reflects many influences and experiences. Prominent amongst these influences is the education that I have received from my patients. Of course a therapeutic professional is required to put away any personal agendas, for fear of subjectively distorting the patient's recovery. A psychiatrist tries to concentrate objectively, but for the purpose of this book it would have been one-sided to include only the observations of my patients' journeys and to completely exclude reference to my own projections. In an authentic description of clinical practice, occasional revelation of the clinician's therapeutic position is informative. This therapy is not rooted in a blank canvas. In order to achieve a balanced description of the reciprocal doctor–patient relationships, I have referenced some of my thoughts and countertransferences whenever it seemed helpful.[2]

Throughout the book, I have made some references to the

standard diagnostic schedule produced by the World Health Organization (WHO) and known as the ICD-10 or the International Statistical Classification of Diseases and Related Health Problems, Tenth Revision. The selected passages are objective agreed descriptors of clinical disorders and their use is part of the standard methodology of psychiatric practice. In psychiatry, diagnosis is not based upon any specific blood test or screen. No such tool exists in mental health care. Categorical diagnosis is useful, and is traditionally seen as a necessary and reliable function within medicine – but it is not sufficient by itself. The diagnoses provide a useful starting point but they are not the full picture, and they may change. What is important is an individual care plan, since people present with varied features of mental distress and some have a mental disorder. Even if diagnostic criteria are met for a particular disorder, two people with the very same diagnostic description can have quite different problems with different severity and distinctive complexity. The recognition of complexity necessitates individual care planning and underpins the person-centred approach to recovery that is the basis of effective care.

All of the recovery stories in this collection are authentic. While they are real (otherwise they would be of no value), the details have been amalgamated and specific identifiers have been altered. Ireland is a small country and it is important to protect the anonymity of anyone who seeks mental health care. It would be wrong to expose those from whom we hope to learn. Over the years, I have always sought the permission of those whose stories I have adapted for teaching (or more recently for broadcasting) and this is true for all the accounts included here. That being said, no character in this volume represents any single private individual, so I wish to assure the reader: anyone who perceives a resemblance to a particular person is mistaken.

There are many reasons why I have included poetry in this book, the most valid being the fact that I regularly use these poems in my own practice. Many of us find it difficult to speak of the mind, and a poem can help to capture a lived experience, adding to it the elusive language of personal reflection, feelings, thoughts and insights. For some of us, an entirely new form of communication is necessary and poetry can be a useful way of introducing this less tangible vocabulary. Mental health care requires an ability to listen and to reflect. Hopefully these poems will provide illustrations of this thoughtful communication and will also provide a way to convey to the reader still unfamiliar with mental health care the ambiguous emotional intensity of a therapeutic relationship.

The heroes of these stories are referred to consistently using the term 'patient' rather than any other descriptor, such as 'service user' or 'client'. In order to avoid being unwieldy, and without striving to be politically correct, it seemed best to stay with a language more familiar to a doctor. Over the past thirty years, my patients have taught me more than can be said and I am very grateful to them. And so the term 'patient' is used as a humane acknowledgement and a universal term signifying one of us who is suffering. To be a patient describes an experience that deserves respect. We will all be patients at some stage and this is part of what it is to be alive.

The Room

My room at St Patrick's University Hospital has a high ceiling, a wooden desk, a bookcase and a number of comfortable soft chairs. To the left of the desk, a tall window looks north to a quiet garden. Beneath the window there is a small side table with bottles of drinking water and some cups. The room is warm and the furniture is reassuringly familiar to me.

The room does not have the iconic psychiatrist's couch. Amongst some books and papers on the desk, there is a computer, a reading lamp and a box of tissues. The floor is covered with a carpet and in front of the desk there is a small rug. In another corner of the room there are two large filing cabinets. A few colourful prints hang on the walls alongside some certificates of qualification. There are many other idiosyncratic bits and pieces; some with personal significance and others with none. There are photos on the bookshelves and toy cars sitting on the desk, as well as some shortbread biscuits, a teapot and a kettle on the side table. There are many books on mental health and history.

Of course, in many ways, none of this really matters. This room could be more or less formal, personal or spartan, but so long as it is a space where people feel able to talk, and feel that someone has listened and heard them, then it is a space of value.

When people come to the room for the first time they are likely to be very apprehensive. Many do not know what to expect. Some may anticipate the dramatic portrayal of mental health assessment seen in popular media such as *The Sopranos* or *Analyse This*. The reality of the psychiatric clinic may turn out to be more prosaic than expected.

Mental health assessment takes more than the right physical setting or the right location. It is hard to define what makes an assessment work, and even harder to ensure that these elements are in place all of the time. In this regard it is helpful to recall the views of Patricia, an especially wise and forthright recovered patient with a capacity for directness. She explained: 'The physical environment for therapy and its quality does matter, of course, but not very much. When you are in distress it's the quality of the care that counts. If you stick the "wrong" people in the "right" office, all you achieve is a nightmare outcome in a nice environment. When I was on the ledge, in the depths of my depression, the most important environmental factors were the ones that empowered me to talk, to feel that someone had listened to me, heard me, and given me hope.'

According to Patricia, it is the quality of the therapeutic relationship that engages recovery. These are the human factors that determine the quality of care. So at any meeting, the priority must be to put the patient at ease, in the hope of building a therapeutic bond. It is good to greet each patient, to shake their hand, to smile, and to offer them a comfortable place to sit and relax, as we prepare to talk and to listen. It is best practice to have read the referral letter in advance and ideally to reread it with each new patient so as to confirm its contents and to establish the facts.

After a brief explanation, a discussion ensues about confidentiality. There are boundaries and limitations with any disclosure and it can be reassuring to understand from the beginning how one's personal information is going to be shared and how it will be used. Sometimes a patient will request to bring a third party into the consultation, at least for a while, and although this may be perfectly reasonable, it is a disclosure and therefore must be informed and consented. Each patient should be in control of his or her own information. This is their right. Their story is their privileged data and it is an intimate marker of their human dignity.

Despite everyone's best efforts, a new patient can be very nervous and may remain uneasy for some time. People do not find it easy to share matters that are painful or private. After a little time, and perhaps a drink of water, most people feel more able to talk freely. Then it is time to seek permission to share information with other professionals involved in the delivery of the care plan – the referring doctor, for instance. Usually patients have no difficulty with this, but it can be reassuring to emphasise that no third party will gain access to the information, without the expressed permission of the patient himself or herself. In truth, what the blood is to a surgeon, clinical information is to the psychiatrist: a psychiatrist must never unwittingly allow the information to spill or to leak.

Just as in any other clinical situation, a psychiatrist is bound by the rules of confidentiality. Nowadays no reputable clinician denies that these rules have limits. There is a balance between the explicit clinical commitment to confidentiality and a clinician's equal responsibility to respect the safety and integrity of others. Confidentiality cannot be a justification for secrecy. It is never legitimate to practise in a way that could place others at risk, and the doctor's commitment to confidentiality does not place the psychiatrist outside the law.

The matters disclosed at the very first meeting or any subsequent ones are likely to be personal, private, intimate and even distressing. In these circumstances a psychiatrist has only one legitimate purpose: to work towards a full understanding of the problems (this is known as 'formulation') and so to develop an agreed plan for care. If at all possible, these meetings should provide relief and support and lead to greater engagement with the therapeutic process and with the recovery plan.

Wherever this type of connection is made, meaningful conversation can begin. With hope, an alliance develops between the person expressing their suffering and the person hearing their pain, and the response is an offering of care. This alliance can occur in the most unexpected of places and at the most unlikely of times.

The therapeutic process comes with certain challenges. It can be difficult for a patient and a psychiatrist or clinician to maintain a therapeutic engagement. A didactic therapeutic position is never helpful. A reciprocal relationship between the patient and the clinician means that an objective therapeutic direction is more likely to be welcomed. With reciprocity, truths about recovery may be shared and may be seen as helpful. In the end, mental recovery is better when it is planned with a human perspective.

We remain social human beings, but today's more atomised life is distressing for some at least. In response to a perceived experience of isolation, a therapeutic relationship with a mental health professional can be useful and even life-saving. But recovery is best maintained where it is supported by friends, and family and community, and when patients can live safely in their neighbourhoods, and where the right to a shared experience of life is cherished.

Recovery is sustained when we can stay healthy, when we can laugh as often as possible, when we can take care of ourselves and ideally take care of someone else as well, and, most of all, when we can be kind to ourselves and to each other. Recovery becomes apparent once we have learned to tame the anxiety of our unconscious mind and choose instead to adapt to life in a more connected and hopeful way.

It seems that once we locate our mind we begin to understand it. The room is a space for the mind, and a metaphor for the mind at the same time. Most of us will never find ourselves on a psychiatrist's couch and yet our lives would be perilous if we did not make space for our mental health. In this space, we can hold up a mirror and acknowledge our search for meaning. By going to the room, life becomes more resourceful and rewarding. In showing up there, we show up for life itself.

Experience

It is difficult to describe depression. Regrettably, many of us think about the D-word as if we shared a common understanding of it, and so we tend to talk about it as if depression had an agreed universal language. In this chapter, three consecutive patients tell their unique stories as they emerged over time, at a series of sessions in my room.

The stories of Carmel, Richard and Liam illustrate distinctive features of mental distress. Each patient had a recognised form of clinical depressive disorder and yet each was entirely different. Each was contemplating suicide when they presented to their doctor. Each had experienced severe distress as well as a personal loss that is often a precipitant of a depressive episode. Sometimes this loss is difficult to account for. Sometimes it is unconscious and sometimes it is difficult to define. Sometimes no stress can be identified because it is obscured and sometimes it is kept secret because it is a source of shame. Whereas grief for the loss of a loved one or sadness at the loss of a much-valued relationship is recognisable and understandable, when loss is not obvious to others, it can be much harder to understand. Sometimes meaningful awareness of depression comes when we least expect it.

Carmel

C armel is a divorced woman with a diagnosis of bipolar mood disorder and related depression.[1] When she first told her doctor her story of depression, Carmel was a college student with her whole life ahead of her. Since that first discussion with her doctor, Carmel has lived thirty years and has had three further serious episodes of what she calls her 'black dog'.[2]

On one occasion, after the birth of her third child, Carmel needed electroconvulsive therapy (ECT), a powerful treatment generally reserved for the most severe mood disorders.[3] Her depressive symptoms have been in remission for some years now. She looks after herself in a way that is conscious of her history of mental disorder but, as she says herself, she is 'not defined or paralysed by it'. She takes regular lithium, which is a natural element – a salt.[4] When it is used appropriately, it is the most effective stabiliser of mood known to medicine.

Carmel's journey towards mental health recovery has not been linear. Much has depended on her individual experience. She is what some like to call an 'expert by experience' and she is an active member of a support group for those with experience of mental health disorder. Every day in Ireland, groups of people meet in neighbourhoods and in towns, hotels and community centres to share their experience of depression with others in search of genuine recovery. Through this fellowship, people find a route to understanding and a source of real hope. At these meetings each story is heard and each hard-earned personal insight is recognised as priceless beyond value. In this emancipating way, organisations such as Aware, Grow, Recovery and AA (and many others like them) probably contribute more to the health of people with mental distress than any official organised service.

When I met Carmel for review she was quite well – and so I asked her to share with me her understanding of her condition. The notes recorded Carmel's diagnosis as bipolar affective (mood) disorder, currently in remission.

Carmel's voice was clear when she talked about her depression. She had considered these issues and had come to views recognisable to many of those who have repeatedly experienced 'the black dog'. She was not boastful about her insight as she explained the conundrum of depression from her point of view.

'My view may not suit everybody but, as I see it, I don't suffer from depression; I experience depression. Between episodes I have a very normal life. My depression is not who I am; it is something that happens to me...

'I certainly get all the problems that you doctors seem to be interested in. When I experience depression I can't enjoy anything and I can't see any hope, my sleep goes and I wake early in the morning, dreading the coming of the day. The only relief is in the evening and then I fear going to bed because I know the whole thing will start all over again. In time, I lose my appetite and my weight falls. My concentration goes and pretty soon I can do nothing. Privately, I have even contemplated death when I have been that down, but luckily I have never done myself any serious harm. I have never lost my reason, but I have been very close.'

Carmel had given thought to the clinical diagnosis of depression and she expanded in a way that had echoes of a common criticism of psychiatry. 'I know you doctors have to do your job, but I want someone to listen to me, not to question me or to be checking lists. I don't want to be let down. When I am depressed, my real experience is feeling alienated and cut off from every one. My real fear is despair and my real pain is indescribable. With help, I have learned that I can get through this and have a good life. Sometimes

I need to find the words to communicate my emotions. I need to have my distress heard.'

Carmel continued: 'I don't want to let down all those people who are like me and who have learned that this experience can be lived through once we work together on a personal recovery plan. We all have to find a way. It is true that lithium works for me and I am sticking to it, but there is a whole lot more to it than that.'

Carmel's view is supported by lots of evidence. Depression is a recurring problem for many people. The uncomfortable truth is that 70 per cent of those who experience a clinical depression will have another depressive illness at some stage. Of those who experience two such illnesses, 90 per cent will have a third. Depression is significant especially when it is profound, pervasive and persistent – and also when other issues complicate it.

In explaining her frustration, Carmel said this: 'Why do we have to wait for months and years sometimes before we do something about these problems? The first time, I was ill for at least eighteen months before I got help. And even then it was another crisis that just forced me to do something about it.'

Carmel had some specific things to say about ECT. 'When I was very unwell, they gave me a course of ECT. I know this might sound odd, but I don't want anyone to disapprove of me for having had ECT. If I am that unwell ever again, I want someone to do as much as possible to get me well again. I know this is a really controversial area and I wouldn't allow doctors to give ECT to those who are unwilling to accept it voluntarily. I would definitely draw the line at that. But with an experience such as depression, we are dealing with serious things. For me, it was as serious as cancer. I wouldn't want someone on the outside banning a treatment like ECT if it's a treatment that has the power to make me well again. The balance of these judgements has to be in my favour. I am the patient. I deserve to have every effective remedy available to me.'

For Carmel, the problem of depression was not just about being afraid to seek help. As she put it to me: 'There is a problem of language as well. When we talk about "depression", we are all talking about different things and there is so much confusion. All I know is what happened to me. The effect of my depression was deep and I could see no way out from a very dark place. Every aspect of my life seemed to be overwhelmed. Since then, the acknowledgement and treatment of my illness has made the difference to my wellness. If I had to sum things up I'd say that depression is an experience I have had more than once, but it is not my life. Luckily, I am able to live by my recovery plan. I can recover fully and stay well.'

Experience

I stepped from plank to plank
　　So slow and cautiously;
The stars about my head I felt,
　　About my feet the sea.

I knew not but the next
　　Would be my final inch, —
This gave me that precarious gait
　　Some call experience.

～

EMILY DICKINSON

Richard

Richard is a quantity surveyor. He had been a postgraduate student in the US and lived there for several years. During the boom years he returned to Ireland, got a high-powered job in the city, married and started a family. Then he decided to move out to the countryside in search of a better quality of life. He joined a small practice in a quiet town, but the anticipated gentle pace of life did not materialise. These were the days when the roar of the Celtic Tiger drowned out all but the most earth-shattering of sounds. Richard found himself trapped in a never-ending cycle of work. He put in longer hours, travelled greater distances from home and felt more and more exhausted. At times, he was so consumed with work that he became alienated from his family and friends.

Suddenly, the bad luck that comes in threes visited Richard: a client sued him for negligence; his fellow partner in the practice decided that he wanted to take early retirement, which meant that Richard would have to buy him out; and a surprise audit by the Revenue Commissioners resulted in a demand for a very large sum of back taxes. Any one of these would be enough to break even the healthiest of people, let alone someone with Richard's pace of life.

Richard's wife had long sensed that something was wrong. He had become increasingly withdrawn and unable to sleep. He got no pleasure from his daily life. His loss of appetite meant that he had lost weight. Sexual intimacy between Richard and his wife had ceased entirely for nearly six months. In distress, Richard's wife brought him to see their GP.

The GP suspected that Richard was depressed but knew that almost any medical illness could be depressing, so it was essential to eliminate as many of these medical diagnoses as possible. All of the clinical investigations on Richard came back with normal results: his physical exam was fine and all tests of his blood, kidney, liver, bone and thyroid function came back within the normal range. There was no evidence to suggest infectious disease or cancer; explanations about his condition were not forthcoming.

Objectively, Richard seemed very downcast and pessimistic. He moved sluggishly and his speech had slowed. It was clear that he was in crisis and suffering from depression.[1] Richard had told his GP that he felt as if he was 'on the ropes', but as far as Richard was concerned all of this was understandable given his circumstances. Richard felt that none of his problems needed intervention from others. The GP had encouraged Richard to attend a counsellor in his local practice and to start a number of sessions of psychotherapy using cognitive behavioural therapy (CBT).[2] He had also advised Richard to consider taking an antidepressant of the SSRI family (selective serotonin reuptake inhibitors).[3] While Richard politely dismissed the counsellor, he vehemently declined the SSRI. At this stage, rather than tell Richard that nothing else could be done, the GP decided to suggest to Richard that he get a second opinion and see a psychiatrist. With his wife's encouragement, Richard reluctantly agreed to come to see me.

During our first meeting, it transpired that Richard's financial position was not as catastrophic as he first thought. His insurers had taken over the negligence claim. It turned out that the tax liabilities related to the years before Richard had joined the practice, so Richard's partner had agreed a settlement with the Revenue Commissioners and had given up any idea of early retirement. With many of the financial pressures resolved, business was better for Richard; however, life was not. Richard could not understand why.

Richard confided that at the worst point of his financial crisis he had felt he was a failure. He was sure that he would lose everything and so he had begun to look at his options. Seeing how little room he had for 'escape', he thought the most attractive option was to die by suicide. He explained: 'I was thinking that my family would get the insurance and that the kids are young, so they would get over it soon enough. My wife would find someone else – hopefully someone who wouldn't let them all down. It seemed like the best way to end the pain and stress I was causing for everyone... But then the business turned the corner and I got over the worst of those feelings. I don't understand why I don't feel better, though.'

A closer questioning revealed a deeper story. As Richard spoke, it became apparent that his problems were of far longer standing. His principal emotion during the past two years had been high anxiety. Sometimes he would suffer sudden crescendos of panic anxiety.[4] 'My heart would pound. I'd sweat and become dizzy. I was sure I was going to die. Now I've got no energy at all. I can't concentrate. When I was younger, I used to be so motivated. I had energy to burn back then.'

I asked Richard if depression and anxiety could be responsible for his tiredness. 'No,' he said, 'I've had enough depression talk from my wife. The truth of it is this: I am not depressed. I am just exhausted. All I need is a good night's sleep and someone to help me to get my energy back. If the GP would give me a sleeping tablet and I could get to the gym I would be all right. It's actually not helpful that people keep interfering and giving me grief about things.'

It was clear that Richard's views were very fixed, but no progress could be made without working within Richard's own understanding of his problems, in the hope of finding some solutions that he could accept. Whether he knew it or not, his emphasis on his loss of energy as a core feature of his problems has a very ancient and august history. For over 2,000 years of medicine, clinicians have described depression or melancholia as a condition characterised by a loss of energy. The clinical features of pervasive sadness and joylessness, guilt and despair were seen, to some extent, as secondary to the loss

of this energetic humour, which was once believed to be essential
to the maintenance of mood and activity. The only language that
Richard could relate to involved an acknowledgement of this key
feature: his lack of energy. He was quite direct: 'My drive has gone.
Somehow I have to get it back. But let's be clear from the start – I
am not going to take any antidepressants.'

Most people experience depression with recognisable forms
of loss. The physical and mental impairments of depression are
so debilitating that their concealment is hard to comprehend and
yet, most of the time, even with this level of distress, depression is
hidden and privately endured.

Richard acknowledged more and more of his problems, but
was adamant that he did not need treatment. However, he decided
that he would keep attending since he found it relieved his distress
to some extent. This was the partnership that we needed to build
upon.

Richard's hesitancy about therapy raises questions about the
values underpinning mental health treatment. While responding to
Richard's dismissal of help, it is hard to ignore the dilemma of the
advocate. Every healer worth their salt wants to heal, but a healer's
desire must be legitimate. For some clinicians, delivery of therapy
merges with their response to the problems of daily living. For this
kind of therapist, mental health disorders are indistinguishable
from ordinary human challenges and so they regard more narrowly
defined medical approaches as lacking an appreciation of holistic
human reality.

Other therapists attempt to transcend the day-to-day issues
and instead see their role as helping people to face the universal
existential reality, which is the inevitability of our death. This
view of therapy celebrates the ultimate achievement of personal
autonomy, the freedom to make choices, to turn away from some
options, and to select sustainable alternatives. When the resulting
psychological outcome is an autonomous one, the therapist regards

this as progress on a journey towards ultimate self-actualisation.

The best approach to mental health care is to place human rights at the heart of any recovery plan. This need not impede practical therapeutic intervention directed towards the 'here and now', especially where the treatment is necessary to sustain life and where therapy is valid in terms of objective evidence. Brief behavioural interventions are focused on problem-solving approaches and they are legitimate when supported by evidence of benefit. In responding to problems such as those experienced by Richard, the therapist's challenge is always to respond in an authentic way; neither to insist on subjective solutions nor to encourage adherence to any one set of personal philosophies. No therapist can claim to have figured out solutions to the universal challenges we all face in life. Our lives are brief and many bogus treatments abound.

Richard might recover by focusing his efforts on addressing the specific challenges arising from his mental distress. If Richard was to fulfil the potential of his life, he needed to get some recovery of his faculties. For better or worse, he needed to regain his functional mental health. Getting personal wisdom or preparation for the existential reality might be done at another time.

In responding to Richard's scepticism, we needed to start by addressing the here and now. Psychological medicine has no role in directing anyone along any specific philosophical route or towards any specific response to the personal challenge of existence. For some people this approach can seem unhelpful, even though it is not intended to be. For Richard, this approach was appealing. In discussing his treatment along these terms, Richard said he felt liberated. With this clarity, he said he felt more engaged. Richard needed to know that no one was about to take over his life. Instead, he was being offered help to revalue that life and regain hope for the restoration of his peace of mind.

During Richard's next sessions the persistence of his depression was very apparent. No straightforward remedy had emerged to dramatically restore his energy levels, and Richard was frustrated by this. In addition, Richard's hostility to the language of mental health made it more difficult to develop a shared understanding.

It seemed that Richard's history was incomplete. Without a full history the psychiatrist is in a very difficult position. There is no specific diagnostic test for clinical depression or anxiety disorder. The diagnosis depends entirely on historical assessment of the behavioural signs and personal symptoms of these common but clandestine problems. Some things had not been said. Perhaps Richard had other details to share that would help us to understand. Maybe there were other things we could consider together on his road to recovery.

Over the coming weeks, Richard revealed more and more. 'I'm the youngest. I've two sisters and one brother. My father died when we were young. That was tough – but I've always just tried to get on with things. I mean, what else can you do?

'I know they say the unexamined life is not worth living, doctor, but the over-examined life is a bit much too. I mean, everyone gets something. I hit a rough patch when I lived in the States, alright. There are times even now when I'd be a bit panicky, but I've always tried to just get on with things.'

Richard's combination of clinical depression and panic anxiety is particularly toxic to recovery. Depression burdens life with past guilt and regrets, but anxiety anticipates life's threats and magnifies them, so that the future becomes full of dread. The combination of depression and anxiety can be paralysing: the sufferer cannot resolve the past, live in the present or prepare for the future.

Panic anxiety disorder frequently coexists with depression and the combination can have a disabling effect on recovery. Panic and anxiety are often accompanied by avoidance behaviour and this is particularly disruptive. Richard was chronically avoidant. He touched on the issue during one of our conversations.

My business partner gets on to me about postponing things at work. Actually, my wife says the same thing at home. I don't think it's a big deal. It's natural enough when you have an awful lot of things on your plate. There's just a lot of responsibility and I don't think it's helped by talking about it. I'm happy to tell my wife about work in the evenings. I'm happy to hear about her work too. But I'm just not one for the endless conversations, you know?'

Richard avoided emotional disclosure and in relationships he feared what he called 'heavy talk'. His history of panic attacks went right back to his early adulthood, and as a result he routinely avoided many circumstances that he felt could precipitate another panic attack. As his mood had deteriorated, he had been avoiding emotional contact more and more. His anxiety amplified his chronic avoidance and this left his life increasingly constricted and limited.

Some of this explained why Richard was less likely to seek help than others with either depression or anxiety problems alone. Even when the anxious depressed do seek help, they are many times less likely to be diagnosed with depression. Anxiety and avoidance tend to mask and postpone the recognition of an underlying melancholy. As a result, the delay between the onset of symptoms and any effective treatment can be many years.

Throughout his presentation, Richard never failed to come to our appointments. His pattern of seeking help while simultaneously rejecting intervention is not at all unusual and he seemed keen to hear about mental health recovery in general. He learned that his experience included symptoms of chaos and panic, loss and despair. We talked about integrated mental health, our shared hope for his recovery and the real prospect of authentic wellbeing and restored balance, but most of all we agreed that his mental recovery was about continuing and going on!

One day, Richard and I spoke about the term 'depression' and he began to talk about his childhood.

'Yes, you could say that there was depression in my family –

although we never really spoke about it. My father died when I was young and I do remember him being very low at times. You know he committed suicide?

'We were on holidays in Wexford when it happened. My father was always fit so it wasn't strange for him to head out early in the day for a swim. I was actually with him that morning. It was very strange. He told me to stay on the beach and he went out swimming. I didn't know what was happening at first and by the time I realised, it was too late. I was screaming on the beach but there was nobody there.

'As far as the coroner was concerned there was no suicide note and there was no other evidence. It was only years after that my mother told me it was definitely suicide. My father had left a note that morning. She hid the note. I think she felt it was her fault.

'I was just angry. I think I got more angry the older I got. I found out that my father had been seeing a psychiatrist – but obviously that was no use to him in the end.'

Richard's personal conclusion was that his father had been depressed, he had been attending a psychiatrist before he died and that no treatment had helped. Likewise, by logical extension, as he saw it, no specific plan could help Richard to cope with his own pain. Most of all, Richard knew that no one had spoken to him as a young man or listened to his anguish in the aftermath of the calamity that turned his family's life upside down. As far as he was concerned, he had been expected to pull himself together when disaster struck and that is what he had always done.

The journey to recovery is a journey through suffering, not around it. No recovery is hastened by trying to escape the pain of depression, but Richard's recovery journey might be made more credible if he was given the power to take steps that he could understand and trust. In a way that he could not recognise, Richard's behaviour was a repetition of the behaviour of his family, including his denial of his symptoms and his rejection of intervention. These had been family features throughout Richard's earlier life. Just as his father's difficulties had been concealed, Richard was concealing and controlling his problem now.

Richard had become trapped in his experience at the expense of the objective potential for his recovery. So far, Richard evaded treatment while still seeming to consider it from a distance. It was as if his recovery was also drifting out to sea. Richard continued to decline treatment. He continued to reject psychotherapy or medication, although he passively tolerated our meetings.

Richard came to two more sessions, during which he did not speak about his father. He wanted to discuss the measures he might take to regain his energy. He felt he had plenty of options, including exercise and a healthier diet. He spoke about the possibility of returning to the States for a new business opportunity.

Towards the end of our last session, Richard seemed to be watching the clock. We spoke about this and he said: 'You know, I've been wondering how I'm supposed to wind this up. It's been really nice talking with you. I'm sure it's been a help. I know my wife's a lot happier that I came here – so I'm sure that means it was the right thing to do!

'Look, there are a few things I need to work on. But I've done it before and I can do it again. I'm certain of that… And I know I could always come back and see you some other time, if I had to. Thanks for your time, doctor. It's been a help. I'm sure it's been a help.'

Late Fragment

And did you get what
you wanted from this life, even so?
I did.
And what did you want?
To call myself beloved, to feel myself
beloved on the earth.

~

RAYMOND CARVER

Liam

Liam is an accountant working in a large firm in the city. He has heavy professional responsibilities. At the height of the Celtic Tiger years, Liam took stock options in lieu of payment and other bonuses. As boom times came to an end, he lost many of these supposed benefits and so he began to work very long hours. He was unaware of his growing distress. What happened next exposed him to a new kind of experience, one that he had never anticipated.

Liam's favourite source of relaxation was cycling and he liked to take part in voluntary events, raising money for charity. One day he was cycling for his local cancer support group when he had an accident. The crash was minor but Liam collapsed immediately afterwards. His wife rushed him to an accident and emergency department where he was briefly admitted to the medical intensive care unit. He was told he had suffered dehydration, although he believed that he had actually come close to dying.

Following tests in the hospital, Liam was discharged. He was told that his brain scan was normal and he was sent home in an apparently healthy state. After a few days at home he appeared to make a reasonable recovery. Then he returned to work, where no one noticed that he had lost much of his old zest and natural enthusiasm. Something was not quite right.

Occasionally depression can have an abrupt onset, which takes everyone by surprise. Curiously abrupt presentations may be easier to resolve than problems that have an insidious or prolonged onset, especially because sudden onset suggests that an acute medical basis is more likely to be a cause.

Initially, Liam's wife regarded his distress as understandable. After all, he had been under very great stress at work since the financial collapse and he had just come through a possible near-death experience. However, as Liam's capacity steadily diminished and his mood fell, his wife began to see that he was suffering more and more. Secretly, Liam had begun to despair. As he lost hope, he began thinking about his 'options'. For the first time in his life it seemed to him that one of these options included taking his own life. He began planning to die by hanging himself.

Why had Liam despaired? His personal dilemma must have been utterly obscure to most people – and it might have remained so but for the incident while cycling. Liam might have remained in a completely private torment. Apart from his experience while cycling, nothing appeared to have happened on the surface. Liam seemed to have no distinctive problems. There were no major health issues. There were no apparent changes to circumstances. Life at home and at work seemed to be going just fine. And yet Liam sought help from his GP and was referred to me.

When I met Liam, he began to describe his problem. He spoke in very hushed tones and he repeatedly requested guarantees of his confidentiality. What emerged from his story came as a complete surprise. Unbeknown to others, Liam had lost his ability to read.

He began to explain. 'I can still read words but I am no longer able to read numbers. You have got to understand the gravity of this. My concentration is completely gone. I can't read numbers – and I live by numbers! I used to be able to race through the *Financial Times* and I could take it all in. Now, everything is in a total jumble. I can't make sense of any of the numbers. I have to be able to do the numbers or I cannot live. Sooner or later I will be found out and I just dread to think what is going to happen then.'

Liam was looking for help. He had no previous history of depression or of self-harm. He was not irrational. In assessing his suicidal risk, it was apparent that there was very little objectively to go on. He promised to give a guarantee of his safety and he agreed that despair was not the answer. 'My death would not address the problem, let alone help anyone else,' he said.

An assessment of suicide risk is a very inexact clinical exercise. There is no specific or reliable test for suicide. No one can reliably predict who will or will not take his or her own life. Neither is there any way of preventing someone who is sufficiently determined or sufficiently unwell from finally completing a suicidal act. This fact is balanced by the reality that suicide is still a rare, although increasingly frequent, act and most commonly it is an act carried out by people who are objectively and measurably unwell.

All psychiatrists are trained in the assessment of suicidal risk but at an individual level these assessments have less predictive value than is sometimes understood. There are a number of recognised clinical correlates for suicidal risk and a psychiatrist is responsible for making this assessment. In practice, doctors rely heavily on the history of harm and the objective evidence of mental disorder. After that, they hope that forming a therapeutic relationship will lead their patient to recovery.

The clinician can often feel very isolated when making judgements on the balance of experience and without substantial objective evidence or reliable data. Sometimes, in retrospect, these estimates seem to have no more validity than those of the financial analyst who observes the market and then makes a judgement as to whether the stock will rise or fall.

Despite this caution, recognised indicators include the presence of clinical depression, a history of previous suicidal behaviour and a family history of death by suicide. Evidence shows that suicide is more common in males than in females and more often completed if these factors are combined with intoxication or the use of violent means, such as firearms. Still, predicting the future is at best an inexact science. No one can tell for sure where or when a tragedy will happen. What matters most of all is the patient's own capacity and commitment to recovery.

Liam had given his guarantee, but objectively there was no certain way of knowing whether in this instance it should be relied upon. The assessment of risk may not be perfect but there is more to building a therapeutic relationship than requesting reiteration of guarantees of safety. Objectively his guarantee was worthwhile, since he had few of the risk correlates described. Together we agreed that his guarantee represented an emblem of his commitment to recovery. This was a commitment we shared.

In the meantime, it was necessary to investigate Liam's specific concerns. His complaint of the inability to read numbers is a rare but recognised symptom of a variety of brain disorders. On clinical examination of his central nervous system, there was no abnormality and so he needed an assessment from one of my colleagues, a neuropsychologist, who was able to assess his mental functions using clinical measures within her expertise. Liam listened to an explanation of all of this as I wrote a detailed letter requesting an urgent neuropsychological assessment and a range of blood tests to rule out a variety of physical illnesses, any one of which could possibly have contributed to his decline. Liam needed to stay off work and he agreed to try to rest. His GP was happy to write a sick note for him and Liam agreed to return to see me soon.

One week later, Liam's blood tests were back and it was clear that he was very unwell. His symptoms were explained. He had succumbed to an unrelated medical disorder that was causing a rare problem for his brain. His thyroid gland had become underactive and antibodies generated from within his body were circulating in his bloodstream and attacking this key hormonal gland. Liam's thyroid function was grossly abnormal and his thyroid antibody titres were very high. In addition to causing hypothyroidism, these same antibodies were cross-reacting and attacking his brain in an acute autoimmune disorder known as Hashimoto's encephalopathy.[1] It was this attack on his brain that was impairing his concentration and causing his specific cognitive disability, mood-related problems and depression.

The neuropsychology report confirmed specific areas of functional deficit underlying Liam's symptoms of anarithmetria (his difficulty with numbers) and my colleague recommended a more detailed brain scan in addition to those carried out in the accident and emergency department weeks before. These new functional images later revealed the specific areas of Liam's brain that were under the immune attack.

Treatment with steroids and immune suppressant drugs rapidly shut down Liam's brain attack. Over some weeks his cognitive ability returned and in particular his facility with numbers was restored. With further correction of his thyroid function, his mood also recovered. Alongside this progress, Liam was able to return to work.

Liam's dramatic illness and his even more dramatic recovery are unusual, but they serve to illustrate some key principles. The acute medical problems Liam had experienced were hidden from everyone because of stigma and fear of mental disorder. In the end, Liam's medical problem came to light because of a chance event. Shame and guilt grew upon the bedrock of his bewilderment and his dread of mental disorder. At one stage his faculties appeared to be disappearing rapidly. What was Liam to think? The 'collapse' event while cycling may have been a preliminary to his real illness, or it may have been a classic 'red herring' to which all the other plausible explanations ultimately gave way. This unforeseen event allowed Liam to seek help and eventually to reveal his secret problem. A full confidential assessment allowed a treatment plan that fully resolved his mental difficulties.

Fortunately, Liam's recovery brought him restoration to full health. In his own words, he was back to his 'old self once again'. But in some ways he believed he had changed too. He saw this 'change' as something to acknowledge as a positive enlightenment, coming in the aftermath of distress and in the wake of recovery.

Liam explained the situation in this way. 'I am fully better but the experience has changed me. I feel as though I have seen into an area of life I imagined I would never be part of. This episode has made me think about things. Before I became ill, I totally overestimated the boom. When I was depressed, I totally overestimated the gloom. Maybe my recovery will be about learning to see things as they really are; neither as a dream or a nightmare.'

The day came when the risk to remain tight in a bud was more painful than the risk it took to blossom.

ANAÏS NIN[2]

Worth

Mental health problems are always in the news. Depression, anxiety and suicide are subjects exposed every day in our local and national media. Sadly, these stories are rarely positive and their human perspective is often lost in the divisive debate about the adequacy of our mental health services. Good news about mental health recovery is in very short supply.

A stigma is a mark, and in the case of mental distress it means any label that discriminates against effective support and treatment.[1] Given our history, stigma – arising from the failure of Irish mental health care – is understandable. Less than fifty years ago, nearly 2 per cent of the Irish population was compulsorily detained in a mental asylum. Psychiatry was commonly associated with large-scale institutionalisation and its therapy was dominated by the prescription of numerous ineffective and often hazardous treatments. Despite huge improvements in mental health services, the Irish consciousness retains many of its stigmatic fears and vivid memories regarding historical mental health care. This memory continues to deter us. Even after three decades of community-based mental health service our faith in recovery is as sceptical as ever. Stigma and self-stigma (the experience of personal shame and guilt arising from one's own mental disorder) are the real enemies of mental health recovery.

Great strides have been made to increase public awareness, knowledge and understanding of mental disorder.[2] Advocacy and awareness campaigns such as See Change have had measurable success, and there has been genuine progress made by the media in their handling of sensitive mental health issues. However, the evidence is that increased awareness alone cannot bring about a change in stigmatic behaviour. Stigma is not an individual issue but a societal one. Evidence from the World Health Organization suggests that overcoming stigma will require cultural change. This must involve everyone, leading to us behaving in a different way towards those with mental distress. In our educated society, levels of mental health literacy are higher than ever and yet mental stigma remains very great. It appears that increasing public information about the brain does not bring about a reduction in stigma. Stigma is not simply a consequence of ignorance. It is a medium of discrimination and injustice. The exclusion of those with mental disorder from our society, from our work places and from our shared neighbourhoods must be seen for what it is: a denial of the human rights of those with mental disorder.

In one way or another, accessing health care remains problematic, but in Ireland when we speak about the challenges of health care policy we tend to avoid the substantive issues, which are actually about quality and standards. As a nation, we have spent years debating the location of health services, with perennial controversy about the survival of local hospitals or the location of cancer services or most recently the location of our national children's hospital. We persist with these arguments about lands and locations but speak little about the standards and quality of our services and their values. As soon as the debate about its location is off the health agenda, we tend to leave the consideration of the content of care to the experts, until we are briefly shocked by revelations regarding derelict clinical behaviours or disheartening outcomes.

In post-Tiger Ireland the pursuit of better standards of service should dominate our health care debate. Lobbyists seeking facilities in one locality or another still preoccupy our health care agenda. Others campaign for services in primary care, and still others promote regional or national centres. If there is ever a clamour regarding improved standards or better clinical outcomes, it tends to be episodic and is not sustained. Without real change in legislation and behaviour the obstacles experienced by those with mental disorder will continue and the spotlight of our collective concern will move rapidly onto other less alienated agenda.

The national strategy for Irish mental health services is known as A Vision for Change. It recommends the ultimate closure of most stand-alone mental hospitals (or 'approved centres' as those inspected by the mental health commission are known). The Vision policy looks to rely for inpatient care on small units attached to general medical hospitals. Comprehensive resources in the community are meant to provide alternatives to hospitalisation, but these community facilities tend to be under-resourced. It is remarkable that the idea of centres of excellence is accepted in cancer care and cardiac care and in almost every area of medicine – but not in mental health. The stigmatic shadow cast by the memory of the asylum is very long.

More than forty years ago it was decided that Irish mental health services should be relocated to the community and should no longer be confined within the old discredited asylums. The decision to move to the community was necessary because of the failure of an asylum system, which was rightly exposed as ineffective and unjust. Public asylum care had expanded for over a century, driven by social desperation and political expediency and without evidence of recovery. Although the twentieth century move to the community was undoubtedly well intentioned, the community has not been well resourced in Ireland. Neglect of mental distress and alienation of those who seek help is still commonplace. Those with a twentieth-century hostility to inpatient care even go so far as to deny the gravity of mental disorder, apart from the most narrowly defined notion of schizophrenia, and so the real range and complexity of service has often been ignored.

In reality the best international models of community mental health care recognise a need for a balanced health care system with a mixture of sources of care. This balanced system functions within a variety of care settings delivering recovery in the community along with specialised inpatient facilities and a highly developed range of expertise where that is required. It is clear from international developments in mental health care that the goal of reducing stigma and improving quality of service will require more than just a policy on relocation of service to the community.

Given their volume, it is not surprising that depression and anxiety disorders are the commonest mental health problems seen in general practice. The World Health Organization (WHO) tells us that depression is the largest contributor to the burden of ill health in Europe, with around 20 million people suffering significantly from depression at present. Depressive disorders and its many related challenges are a huge problem for Irish society. Four of the six leading causes of years lived with disability are due to mental health disorders. These are depression, alcohol dependence, schizophrenia and bipolar mood disorder.

In this era of community care, mental disorder remains hidden. Individuals experiencing it remain invisible so that life with mental distress is typically a clandestine experience. Arguably, it is as obscured from our view as it was when so many people were physically hidden behind asylum walls. The inequality of our society has a great deal to do with this invisibility. The likelihood of being unemployed is trebled by the fact of having a mental disorder. The poor and the marginalised in Irish life disproportionally use the public mental health services so that to some observers mental disorder has simply become a marker of inequality and poverty. It is true that all health burdens are exacerbated by social inequality, but major mental illness emerges wherever it will. Stigmatic exclusion due to mental distress is experienced universally as human beings in common. It is a problem for those with money and those without, and all those who experience it are discriminated against in countless practical ways.

All groups in society experience a disincentive when it comes to accessing good mental health care. If stigma was an economic issue alone, exclusion would be experienced by the poor alone; in reality, all those with mental disorder experience alienation and discrimination. Identifying mental health stigma as an issue for the poor allows the more comfortably off to remain complacent about it, until it strikes at their own door.

Stigma and self-stigma is the real reason why only a minority of those with mental disorders ever seek professional help. The decision to come to see a psychiatrist is never taken lightly and too often it is a decision that is made very late. One in five of us will have a depressive illness in our lifetime and yet most of our mental health issues are neglected for decades. Each person has their own view about depression and their own understanding of what it is to be depressed. The variety of attitudes and their subjectivity makes the challenge of taking coherent action for mental health all the more difficult. However, the injustice experienced by people with mental disorder means that people are genuinely afraid to seek help. Stigma is a cultural issue – and people in our culture feel that by getting help they will be making matters worse in many ways. Stigmatic consequences for insurance, housing and employment represent real obstacles to recovery for those who experience a mental disorder.

In 2013 St Patrick's Mental Health Services published some disturbing findings from its own nationwide survey of attitudes to mental health disorder in Ireland. Over one-fifth of people surveyed believed that those suffering from mental health problems are below average intelligence and 31 per cent of respondents revealed that they would not accept someone with a mental health disorder as a close friend. It was discovered that 62 per cent would discriminate against hiring someone with a history of mental illness on the grounds that they would be unreliable, and 42 per cent believed that undergoing treatment for a mental health disorder is a sign of personal failure. As Paul Gilligan, CEO of St Patrick's, stated at the time of the release of this data: 'A lack of understanding of mental health problems is still fuelling stigma and preventing people from accessing support.'

Arguably, once people are in a system their care will be satisfactory; but commonly the required assessment is denied or delayed for years or even for decades. From anxiety disorders to mood disorders, the length of time between the onset of symptoms and obtaining professional help is often more than ten years. During this delay the risks to the individual and the losses to society are very great. The reality is that, with effective intervention, problems are eminently treatable.

Alyson

lyson is a 32-year-old woman from Co. Cavan. She has been married for nearly four years to David and they live on a farm of 90 acres. They have no children. Alyson asked her GP for a referral since she felt very low in mood and was finding it more and more difficult to cope. Alyson's GP had tried to assess and treat her within his clinic and he wanted to refer her to the counsellor in his practice, but Alyson declined. She explained that she didn't want to see anyone locally because people might talk: 'It's a tight-knit community where I live – but I don't want everybody knowing my private affairs.'

Alyson said that her mood had been very low for the previous three months, but as we talked it became clear that her loss of joy and her sense of despair had been present for much longer, maybe even for six months. Recently, she had contemplated ending her life and she felt profound guilt about this hopeless feeling.

As a teenager, Alyson had overcome similar episodes with the support of her family and the help of her GP.[1] At that time she had also been cutting herself on the arms.

'I had a few low points in my teens – one bad patch in particular. Everyone became very concerned once they found out I was cutting myself. But they didn't seem to understand that I was doing it out of frustration and not out of any real wish to kill myself.

'This time around, I haven't done anything risky or self-destructive. I can see that that kind of behaviour in the past got in the way of any real help because everybody around me just started to freak out. I feel very hopeless at this point. But I'm not going to do anything to harm myself. I really just want to be well again.

That's why I'm here.'

It was clear that Alyson's thinking was not persecuted and she was not deluded in any way. Her worries about privacy were not based on any irrational beliefs. Her sense of reality was not impaired, even though she was very pessimistic and sceptical. She blamed no one else for her misery. According to Alyson, the facts were clear.

'I can't have people intruding on my personal business. People never trust you again if they find out that you have mental health problems. If I lose that trust I'll never get it back. People will always look at me differently.'

It was clear that Alyson's views were full of a personal sense of stigma, but this was not the time to try and dissuade her. My job was to listen, to form a correct diagnosis and to work with Alyson. She had come looking for help and she insisted she wanted to work on an effective treatment plan. She was fluent and forthright, but she had very little good to say about herself.

'I just feel so unattractive and so overweight. My skin is terrible and it is getting worse all the time. I have pustular acne, and now I am getting facial hair as well. It's embarrassing.

'The physical end of things is terrible – but it's really tough emotionally as well. I feel so guilty about my depression. I know it's having a terrible effect on David. He is a good man and he is walking on eggshells around me. He is always afraid of saying or doing something that might make it worse. It is nonsense, of course: none of this has anything to do with him.

'I'm beginning to wonder about our future. I look at myself sometimes and I can't fathom how he stays with me. What on earth could he see in me?'

Low self-esteem is a common feature of depressive states but when self-deprecation is persistent it is more helpful to see it as a predisposing risk factor to depressive episodes rather than a feature of a depression. Chronic low self-esteem makes depression more likely. Persistently poor self-regard may be a risk factor for further depression.

Alyson explained that she hadn't always felt this way. There had been times when she felt more confident about herself, more content with her appearance and more sure of her own ability. 'There were times,' she said, 'but all of that seems a distant memory now.'

Alyson talked about her family. 'My parents have both passed away. My father was a factory worker who died young enough. Heart attack. My mother used to work as a care assistant in the local hospital and she died two years ago. Breast cancer.

'Dad was a drinker – a heavy drinker. I wouldn't describe him as an alcoholic or anything, and he was a decent man. I've two siblings. We all get along well but I wouldn't divulge too much personal stuff with them.'

Alyson was hesitant when talking about her life and describing the circumstances she had lived through. Gradually, she relaxed and spoke more openly about her history and about her present circumstances.

'I find that my concentration is affected recently. Even the simplest task fazes me. I feel like I can't get anything done. Everything seems to be a mountain to sort out. I feel sad, alright, but mostly I feel drained. I'm tired of all of this.

'Every day it's the same thing. I wake up early and my heart is beating so loudly that I think it's going to burst out of my chest. I feel afraid before the day ever starts. And it just gets worse as the day goes on. There's this feeling of dread. It's not even about anything in particular. "Nameless dread." That's how I would describe it.'

Although objectively Alyson looked perfectly presentable, she was still very self-conscious about her appearance, her poor skin and her obvious acne. Her dark facial hair embarrassed her.

'I feel so bad about the way I look. My skin is getting worse, and because my hair is very dark I have to go for electrolysis to get rid of it. Lately I have stopped bothering to take care of myself. I eat for comfort and mostly in the evenings – often if David is out working. I used to exercise to shift my weight but now my energy is so low that I can't get myself going to do anything. I feel really negative about the way I am. I can't concentrate or get motivated. It's as if my thinking has just slowed up.'

Alyson agreed to answer some direct questions. Although these would be about personal and private matters, she said she understood their purpose and she didn't mind answering. In response, she stated that she was not binge eating, self-starving or purging. She explained that her periods had become 'non-existent'. In the past they had been painful and associated with lots of distress, especially for the week beforehand.

'I could be like an antichrist for a few days and then wonder looking back on it what it was all about. My periods were irregular but now they are very infrequent. David says I have given up on us having children together. In reality, my head is too wrecked. And anyway, I have no desire for sex. Of course, I feel guilty about that as well.'

Alyson described her lifestyle in more detail. 'I'm not a big drinker but I do smoke: twenty a day. I've never used drugs. I'm not a fan of prescribed drugs either, by the way. I've never had any major medical problems, really. My GP has spoken to me about my weight. He says it's a concern. He thinks I'm at risk of diabetes at this stage. I told him I need to be better before I can think about my general health, but it's probably just an excuse. To be honest, I don't feel I have it in me to do anything about my weight now. I'm really ashamed about it. I wouldn't know where to start.'

We talked more about Alyson's family and her early life. 'No, I wouldn't say anyone in the family had mental health problems. As far as I know, my parents were never ill that way. Looking back now, life can't have been easy for my mother because of my father's drinking. I'd say she must have had a hard time, but in those days no one said anything about that sort of thing. Overall, I'd say they were as happy as most people.'

When we talked about Alyson's self-harm during teenage years she became more distressed. 'I was just a very mixed up young girl. I had no idea what a fuss would be made of it. People started presuming that I must have been neglected or sexually abused, which was an appalling suggestion to me. When I wouldn't go along with that suggestion they seemed to imply that I was hiding something or must have had something else wrong with me. In the end they said I had a problem with my personality. They said I was emotionally unstable and I was so offended that I decided I was never going back to them.[2] In any case they were of no help to me, and somehow I just had to get through a really stressful patch. No one recognised that I was being bullied at school about my weight. I had no one to really support me until I met David.'

It was no surprise to hear that Alyson had suffered an earlier episode of depression. Three-quarters of adult mental health problems begin before the age of 24. That is why early and effective intervention in adolescence is so important to prevent the development of most adult mental health problems. Self-destructive behaviours are commonly seen in young people with mental health distress. Where this has been a longstanding and characteristic response to stress, it is regarded as an unhelpful maladaptive behaviour and this observation may form part of a diagnosis of personality disorder. It is important to note that these diagnoses have very little validity unless they are corroborated by a history from others with a long-standing knowledge of the patient or unless they are based on detailed and prolonged observation. The diagnosis of personality disorder in adolescence needs to be made at a time other than the moment of acute distress, since the immediate problem can colour the longer-term view.

'Personality disorder' is a term describing a recognisable set of unhelpful characteristics that present before adolescence and persist throughout adult life. It is unwise to make a diagnosis of personality disorder in an acute crisis. The area of diagnosis around personality is one of the least robust or reliable structures within routine adult mental health assessment. Sadly, it is invoked all too frequently and without sufficient corroboration. The result is frequently experienced by the patient as a form of dismissal from mental health care, since patients with these problems are not regarded as responsive to standard treatments.

Certainly, Alyson felt she had been dismissed. This may have been her perception but she told me she was doubly offended by the suggestion that she had something to hide. 'I am not a victim. I have nothing to hide and no one has ever abused me.'

On the evidence of her history so far, Alyson had number of possible diagnoses. Firstly, Alyson did reach criteria for a diagnosis of recurrent depressive disorder – but she did not have a personality disorder. It would be necessary to address her recurring depressive episodes and together we would outline the elements of a therapeutic plan.

Secondly, we agreed her overweight was clinically significant for a number of reasons. Overweight could be a perpetuating factor for her low mood and for her poor self-esteem, but it was possibly even more significant because of her risk of developing diabetes. She was a smoker and this was a concern for her physical health as well as her mental health. The combination of diabetes and smoking is particularly toxic for the heart and circulation, as it leaves people at greater risk of damage to their blood vessels both large and small, with increased risks of heart attack or strokes.

Thirdly, her history also suggested that she could be suffering from another common hormonal problem called polycystic ovarian syndrome (PCOS) and this might be the underlying hormonal explanation for many of her disfiguring problems, including her acne and her facial hair.

All of these problems would need deeper investigation and

further clarification but they were amenable to treatment. It was essential to offer Alyson the hope of recovery and the full expectation of wellness. Of course, this information was quite a lot to take in. Many people feel distressed when they hear their diagnosis for the first time and so it was not surprising that Alyson responded with dismay.

'With all due respect, I didn't plan on coming here for a whole review of my health. Yes, I expected you to diagnose my depression and maybe confidentially recommend a counsellor – but that was it. Now I feel like I am getting the third degree from you. I didn't expect you were going to tell me off about my weight and my smoking.'

What should a doctor do at this stage? The last thing anyone would want to do is argue with Alyson. No one in distress is ever convinced by an argument, no matter how compelling its objective logic might seem. Alyson's response was another form of stigma, the common belief that mental health is separate from general physical health. While we are frequently inclined to see mental health as different from physical health, this distinction is actually false. There is no division between the brain and the rest of the body. I was sorry that Alyson felt offended and, in the face of her stigmatic reaction, the only course was to listen and to try to offer hope. Hopeful listening is the best way forward.

Alyson had mentioned that she expected to be recommended a counsellor, so one response was to agree that a counsellor would be a very good way to proceed. Part of my task was to introduce Alyson to the team of professionals most likely to have the skills needed to help her with her recovery plan. This would have to proceed at whatever pace was acceptable to Alyson.

Alyson would need counselling and possibly more indepth psychotherapy. A learning-based approach of cognitive behavioural therapy (CBT) was sensible, but she would also need investigation for prediabetes, along with tests for PCOS. This meant a number of blood tests and an ultrasound image of her abdomen in order to visualise her ovaries.

It was clear that Alyson would need support with motivation for weight reduction and smoking cessation, in order to return to normal weight and general fitness. She may also need some medication. The best way to deliver all of this was to involve a team of professionals working together with Alyson to resolve her problems. The initial team would include her GP, a psychotherapist, a gynaecologist and myself. Coordinating this team was one task. Maintaining Alyson's engagement throughout would be the greater challenge.

The hope was that Alyson would allow the investigations, blood tests and ultrasound to be arranged through her GP, and that she would agree to start seeing a counselling psychotherapist for some CBT. We could review the progress in a few weeks' time when her results were back and after she had time to ponder all she had heard. The main task was to encourage Alyson to come back, to engage her in a plan for her care and to help her to see all of this as a positive process, with a necessary set of steps leading towards the restoration of her whole physical and mental health.

Some weeks later Alyson returned to my room. This time she brought her partner, David, with her and she asked that I would see them together. By now we had the results of her blood tests and ultrasound, which her GP had arranged in the local hospital. It turned out that Alyson did not have diabetes, but the tests had confirmed the diagnosis of PCOS.

On learning about the diagnosis, Alyson had begun researching online. She had gathered some information on PCOS from the National Library of Medicine in the US.[3] Together we read through this information and Alyson asked for clarifications as we went along.

Alyson and David had already been to see their GP and he had given them plenty of information on the treatment options for PCOS. We discussed all of this in detail. Raised cholesterol and prediabetes are common with PCOS, which emphasised the need for Alyson to make changes to her lifestyle. There is no single cure for PCOS, but early intervention and management is necessary. The most important intervention would be lifestyle change, since improved diet and exercise are shown to be beneficial. The evidence is that a reduction in weight of even 10 per cent can restore normal ovulation and regular periods. The risk of heart disease would be greatly reduced for Alyson if she could stop smoking. Regular monitoring of blood pressure, cholesterol and blood sugar would be essential also.

During this discussion, Alyson was very forthcoming. 'I do want to feel better physically. It seems right to have some more gynaecological assessments – because David and I are worried about fertility. I am clear about the health risks that come with my weight. I'll see how the weight loss goes. And if I can't help the PCOS that way, I suppose I can think about some medications that might work. Maybe. I have loads of information now, but I suppose the main question is this. What, if anything, has all of this got to do with my mental health?'

The answer is that mental health and physical health are all connected. Depression is a hormonal disorder – so too is PCOS. Alyson's diagnosis reminded me again about the need for an individual assessment in patients who report depression and anxiety. Her story also illustrates the fact that mind and body are one whole being. Taking care of one aspect is inevitably good for the other. Alyson was less than convinced by these views but she did credit the progress that had been made since we had first met. We persisted together.

Depression always has a context. In Alyson's case, the growing frustration she felt with her life was reminiscent of her childhood experience. The prospect of recovery would only become truly real when an authentic plan was in place. It was not going to be easy for Alyson to give up smoking, take more exercise and lose weight. There were challenges ahead, but Alyson did agree that an experienced psychotherapist could offer worthwhile support. It was important that Alyson regain her sense of self-worth.

David remained quietly attentive throughout most of this session. Then I asked him how Alyson's diagnosis would affect him. 'Well…it's good to have an answer, anyway. Alyson's been really unhappy and I've been worried about her. I'm just not sure how all this is going to get done. I thought she'd come here and it'd be more straightforward. I was thinking you'd prescribe an antidepressant and that would be that.'

At this point, Alyson interrupted. 'David, you sound just like my family when I was younger! You just want me "fixed". Sometimes I think you're the one who's ashamed. Sure, it'd be great if the doctor could just give us some magic tablet that would do the trick. But we all know that's not going to happen. There's a lot more to it than that.'

Alyson then spoke to me: 'I do want to work on my weight. And I want to try to stop smoking. I would like a counsellor and maybe you could recommend someone. I still don't want anyone local for that. Maybe you think that is foolish, but I have to be clear with you on that.'

Alyson had begun her journey to recovery and she did made great progress over the following year. To date, she has lost nearly 20 kg and she is still off cigarettes. Her blood pressure is normal and her cholesterol levels are coming down. She continues to see her local GP and she has been to a counsellor about eight times.

The last time I saw Alyson, she had this to say: 'So much has changed. I've learned a lot from my medical check-ups – my GP has been good. The weight loss feels nice and I love being off the cigarettes. I feel like I can really trust my counsellor – she's been so kind and she's discreet. It's actually hard to say which part of the plan has been the most helpful. I'm sure one thing helps another. I have had tough days, but I'm definitely going in the right direction. And David has been great. We are getting on better with life and he is being supportive. Maybe I was unkind that day when I said he was ashamed of me. He has actually always been there for me, even when we were first together. Whenever I've been down, he has been really patient – and I know that's not easy. In fairness, David has had his own tough times too. Somehow I believe that we will work things out differently now that I am getting well. We could have a really interesting future ahead of us.'

With a Flower

I hide myself within my flower,
That wearing on your breast,
You, unsuspecting, wear me too—
And angels know the rest.

I hide myself within my flower,
That, fading from your vase,
You, unsuspecting, feel for me
Almost a loneliness.

∿

EMILY DICKINSON

Freedom

People recover every day, but most of us in modern Ireland do not believe this is so. It seems that our societal attitude to mental distress lacks sufficient hope. There are many reasons for this, but one of these must surely be a denial of the potential value of mental health treatment.

When I started out in training as a young psychiatrist I remember wondering whether I would be able to sustain the optimism needed to maintain a life working in mental health care. I started to worry that my patients might depress me. Without knowing it, I had succumbed to of one of the oldest stigmatic fears: the belief that mental illness is contagious. The truth is that mental disorder is not 'catching'. You cannot just 'pick it up somewhere'. As with any other cause of ill health, it has a basis which goes beyond these misunderstandings and which is readily available to study and can be understood.

Our collective pessimism about recovery endures despite the growing evidence of effective psychotherapies, skilled professional teams and new therapeutic supports. If mental health care were perceived as worthwhile, would more people seek recovery? Would more of us demand effective help and insist on less delay? Is it possible that our pessimism endures because of ignorance about recovery? Or does it say something about our fear of losing control?

My first post in Ireland as a consultant psychiatrist was with the health service executive (HSE) at a large general hospital in Dublin. It may seem curious that a psychiatrist should spend so much time working in the emergency department (A&E), but it turns out that this is the place where many people first encounter a psychiatrist.

When crisis and calamity strike, people find themselves in the emergency department. Of course, the busy casualty department is not an ideal setting for psychiatric assessment – but we must make space for each other wherever we can.

The mental health issues appearing in the emergency department are usually those that come to attention only when life goes suddenly out of control. These acute presentations of mental distress are most commonly with deliberate self-harm or episodes of self-poisoning. Through an assessment in the emergency department it frequently becomes clear that this self-harm is a manifestation of a personal crisis – an act of desperation, certainly, but not necessarily a presentation of mental disorder.

By comparison with everyday distress, mental disorder is relatively uncommon. Distress at some stage is universal. All of us have problems, but the experiences of people in crisis vary widely. In the emergency department, self-harm is most commonly recognised as a reaction to life stress rather than a signal of any specific mental disorder. In contrast to these presentations of distress, which are non-specific, presentations of mental disorder have well-defined characteristics and these are open to rigorous diagnostic assessment. Of course the two phenomena do overlap, and mental problems and personal crises frequently coexist. But when these challenges are associated with a fear of losing control, the nature of the real problem is often concealed.

Colm

Colm is a barber. He has a wife, a family, a home and a business. On the surface his life is pretty good. In many respects he is a tidy man. For example, he likes to take care of his own clothes. One day, while carefully ironing his shirt, he accidentally burned his left forearm. The burn was so painful that it required him to go to the emergency department. There his injury was dressed and later he was discharged home.

The very next day, Colm returned to the same emergency department. This time he had a similar injury on his right forearm. This second burn mirrored exactly the original burn on his left arm. The emergency department nurses were at a loss to explain why any man should present to them on consecutive days with symmetrical self-inflicted burns to both of his forearms. At first Colm would not explain it, but with a little persuasion he agreed to stay to speak to a psychiatrist and so I was called to see him.

Colm spoke carefully as we sat in a noisy little side room down a corridor in the emergency department. The busy sounds of activity in the hospital made it hard to find space for reflection, but Colm was keen to speak.

'It's actually a relief to be here and to be talking with you. I've been under quite a bit of stress. Business is not great. One of my kids has been unwell and we're trying to get to the root of what has caused that. I know my wife has been worrying about me a lot.'

So how had he come to injure himself? How had it happened twice? Could he see that it was puzzling? Was he a risk to himself? Was he feeling despair?

Colm denied any real risk to his safety. 'I am not going to harm myself,' he said. 'I never intended to end my life. This is about something else entirely.

'It's hard to find the exact words. All I can say is that my life is becoming chaotic. I'm having a lot of unwelcome thoughts. Images come into my mind – some of filth and contamination. I can't tell anybody about them. I don't call these images up. They just seem to come from somewhere. I find them intrusive. They make me deeply uncomfortable.

'I try to put the bad thoughts out of my mind. Some of them are disgusting. They're all pointless, but they come into my mind despite my best efforts. They go around and around my mind, seemingly without end. I can't clear them. As hard as I try, I cannot put them out of my mind.'

Colm explained his history of similar thoughts. 'I have had bouts of this before and I've been able to get relief by counting numbers in my head. I can place things in order all around me and that seems to relieve things and distract me.[1] I find that if I can place things in straight lines and I can put things in balance all around me, the bad thoughts are contained. I like it when things are in order.

'When my numbers add up and things are where they should be, I feel everything is going to be all right. The terrible horrors that fill my thoughts seem less likely once I can straighten everything out. Does that make sense?'

On closer questioning, it became clear that Colm's mood had been very low for the past three months. 'I'm not sleeping great. I can't say that I'm enjoying much in life. I don't have a lot of energy. I've lost my libido. I can't explain why. I haven't had any intimacy with my wife in some time.

'I have lost interest in lots of things. I'm becoming quite sad – hopeless, actually. It's been going on for a few months now. Initially, I tried sticking to the old plan of counting things and putting things in order. But it doesn't seem to work any more.'

Colm insisted his first injury was probably an unfortunate

accident. However, on reflection, he agreed the second injury had definitely not been by chance. Colm was obsessional about symmetry. Placing things in order and balance usually helped him to dismiss the thoughts of contamination and disaster that were revolving in his mind.

'I know it sounds weird but I'm finding it increasingly difficult to tolerate any lack of symmetry. If things aren't in order I can't drown out my bad thoughts. I think that's why I burned myself. The pain of the second burn wasn't as distressing to me as the asymmetry of having that first burn by itself. I know it must sound like a weird solution, to burn myself like that in order to calm down. But the situation was compelling.

'The symmetry thing doesn't always bother me. When I'm in better form, I can cope quite well with things being all over the place. I'm not always fussy. Believe it or not, when I'm well I can take symmetry or leave it. It's not always a big deal. But lately I haven't been feeling great. Actually, I've been feeling quite low. This has happened a few times before in the past. And whenever it does, the symmetry thing really starts to dominate my mind. There is a part of my mind that thinks that if I get things in line and get things in order, then I'll be able to banish the bad thoughts. That's how it has played out in the past. Every time my problem signs itself in, it uses the same signature.'

Aaron Beck, the father of cognitive behavioural therapy (CBT), coined the term 'logical errors of thinking' to describe the toxic reasoning inherent to the mindset of many depressed people. Beck recognised the negative content of depressive ideas was not just secondary to depressed mood; he saw that negative thoughts were active in perpetuating it. His school of psychotherapy saw these errors of thinking as causative and instrumental in generating the depressive distress. Beck's thesis has since been put to the test and years of rigorous research have confirmed and extended his hypothesis. Depressive thinking can be learned and unlearned.

Colm's mood was responsive to treatment with CBT. This learning therapy is effective and safe. It works by facilitating new thinking and new behaviour and this leads to actual brain change. 'Logical errors of thinking' are unlearned through exposure to real circumstances and they are replaced with constructive reasoning. Colm had some sessions one-to-one with a psychologist trained in CBT.

Colm would be well. With recovery, he regained his sense of wellbeing and his thinking ceased to be magical and superstitious. He began to understand that his depression brought with it obsessive anxiety and compulsive behaviour. Once his mood was restored he was able to relax and to 'go with the flow'. He agreed to work on a treatment plan. His diagnosis was recurrent depression with obsessive-compulsive features. Together we worked on a psychological as well as biological understanding of his problem. As time went on, Colm came to a greater understanding of his own history. 'My mother had depression and I have always been a worrier.'

One day Colm said something that revealed the great distance he had come on his recovery journey. 'Do you know what? I think I am actually getting the hang of this. I am beginning to understand what all of you are really saying to me. It's like this, isn't it? I will be all right just as soon as I am happy to get it all wrong.'

What did Colm mean by this apparent oxymoron? Although his therapist might not have put it to him in so many words, Colm had captured a personal insight and an understanding that would be key to his recovery. He was beginning to see that he needed to abandon his magical and compulsive defence mechanism. His compulsive placing of things in symmetrical patterns was an unsustainable magical defence against his real-life stress. His compulsive behaviour gave him a comforting illusion of control. In the past, symmetry did not just feel right for Colm: it magically prevented life's dangers from coming to him.

When he could be happy with asymmetry (and that had previously appeared to him to be wrong), he would be on the right road to recovery. Colm had other compulsions, including preoccupation with neatness, order and cleanliness. Once he could be happy to give up control over these issues, he could be contented even in a world gone 'wrong'. He would be on the right road. Once he was able to give up the illusion of control he could begin to face the real problems in his life and stop compulsively running away.

Alongside his therapy, Colm agreed to take a selective serotonin reuptake inhibitor (SSRI). These are effective anti-obsessional antidepressants and for many OCD patients they are particularly beneficial. This is especially true in depressed states with obsessional anxiety. He agreed to take the medication every morning. Over the following three weeks at home, his mood lifted and his OCD anxiety reduced. He told me he had experienced a few side effects.[2]

'Initially, I was nauseous but then that passed after a few days. My sleep improved really quickly, which was a great relief. But I notice that I'm sweating at night and this really bothers me. Also, in the mornings I wake up feeling tired.'

We agreed to take some practical steps to overcome these side effects. Since Colm's medication was sedating him, we reversed the usual advice of taking it once daily in the morning and instead he agreed to take it once daily before bedtime. For his mornings, we planned a new routine and Colm was willing to follow this new regimen. From now on, once he awoke in the morning he would get up immediately without delay and go into the shower. With this commitment we worked on a new pattern. Colm would rise promptly when he awoke each morning, doing so regardless of how tired he felt. Colm had a great way of describing this new plan: 'Eyes open – feet on the floor!'

We talked at length about the balance of benefits of the medication over its side effects. Colm was quite clear that he was much better on the medication and in time he felt intense relief from his obsessional anxiety and his compulsive behaviour. His mood had lifted and he was better able to face the challenges of his day. There were still questions to answer if he were to remain well and to avoid the relapsing picture that had become characteristic of his OCD disorder. We were determined things would have to be different this time.

Colm agreed to place a greater value on his recovery. Being well is a great prize. Health is not about being off treatment. A healthy life is one that re-engages with the world, with living, working and loving.

Our recovery mantra was this: 'The plan that gets you well is the plan that keeps you well.' For many people with mental problems, it is the sustainability of the recovery plan that presents greatest difficulty. Getting well is the first issue. Staying well is another challenge. Colm's long-standing compulsive behaviours took some time to resolve. We continued to work on learning new ways of thinking. Colm began to see that his obsessional concerns and logical errors were coming from his brain and that they could be overcome. He began to really believe that there was more to him than this problem.

Obsessional patients can be tormented with thoughts or images that are utterly contrary to their true nature. The most gentle may have ideas of violence, the well behaved may have images of anarchy, and the most appropriate may be tormented with antisocial thoughts. These are doubly distressing because their content is typically full of violence or contamination or offensive sex and because thoughts such as these are completely contrary to the nature of the person themselves.

In response to intrusions such as these, Colm's thinking displayed an obsessional phenomenon called 'magical fantasy'. Many of us think in a magical and superstitious way and in health this is no more harmful than wishing; but in distress, magical fantasy may be the forgotten key to the understanding of obsessive-compulsive disorders. Magical fantasy occurs in response to intrusive thoughts that are ego-alien (thoughts that are contrary to the true nature of the individual) and offers a way of undoing them through compulsive ritual behaviour. Tipping, counting and ritual washing or checking appear to undo the distress of dreaded thoughts especially when these unwelcome ideas are contrary to the self-image of the patient. Unfortunately, magical fantasy is an escape and it can be destructive. Fantasy can temporarily reduce distress but it does so at the risk of turning life into a chess game in which people and events are just pawns whose every move takes on a powerful and yet unsatisfactory significance.

Those who are suffering in this way usually welcome any behaviour that mitigates these ideas and images. We are all familiar with the idea of the compulsive hand-washer. The iconic image of Lady Macbeth is one example. As she tries to distance herself from the king's murder, she repeatedly washes her hands and cries: 'Out – damned spot!' The attraction of this repetitive behaviour is increased since it wards off dreaded thoughts and diminishes fantastic obsessional horrors, as if by magic.

The effect of OCD behaviour upon relationships is also destructive, when human feeling and social interaction is subordinated to the overriding demands of OCD anxiety. Like any addiction, the priority for the person with obsessive-compulsive anxiety is to meet the demands of their distress even if this is at the expense of the human quality of a relationship. This challenge may be particularly distressing for families where one member has OCD. Families often ask, 'What should we do if our son or daughter is insisting on checking or counting before we do anything together?' There is no easy answer to this question. The best way forward is to continue to do ordinary things and to resist the temptation to appease the demands of OCD. When faced with the choice between meeting the OCD demand and doing the ordinary everyday thing, the plan is to resist doing OCD. Appeasement and reassurance are as toxic in OCD as having a row about the issue.

Colm and I met again one day near the end of his therapy. At this stage he had completed ten sessions with his therapist. He told me how that had been going.

'I am much better now since I am able to focus on other things. My priorities have changed in some ways. You know, I used to have to iron my shirts so neatly that they would look just like they first came out of the shop packet – all folded and starched. Now I iron them without folding them and I just leave them hanging on hangers. I am hoping that soon I won't care about ironing them at all!'

In our sessions, Colm and I spoke earnestly about his risks of relapse. He explained the challenges.

'Yes, I've been here before. In the past, I haven't really stuck with any treatment plan. I know now that I need to keep going with this. It's like we keep saying: "The plan that gets you well is the plan that keeps you well." I know from my past experience that ignoring these things doesn't help. I am happy with the plan we have. I do worry about the medication sometimes. I feel well on it and we've found ways around any of the side effects I was having at the start. But how can I be sure that I'm not going to become completely dependent on the medication? Or what happens if I start to become immune to it?'

Colm's fears were completely understandable, but the facts are these. Antidepressants are not addictive. Unlike benzodiazepines and sedatives, they do not lead to dependency.[3] Neither do they 'wear out' or lose their potency. They are effective and safe when used under proper supervision.

We discussed Colm's ambivalence about his psychological and chemical treatment at one of our later sessions. Colm wanted to know the facts. According to the best guidelines, a single episode of major depression warrants continued treatment for at least nine months after recovery. Early cessation of therapy invites relapse.

Colm had a recurring depressive illness and so he needed to consider the benefits of taking long-term treatment.

Colm had relatively few side effects to worry about. He had no sexual side effects. Unlike nearly 20 per cent of people on SSRIs, he had not lost his libido and he had no ejaculatory failure. He experienced some sweating and nausea at first and he was a little more tired when on the medication, but overall it agreed with him. Despite this, Colm had concerns.

'Really, the side effects are mild enough. It's not the side effects that bother me. It's just the fact of being on the medication that gets to me. I somehow feel that I should not have to be on the tablets. I don't even take an aspirin! I have found it hard to accept being on medication every day. I know that the treatment is working. But there's something about accepting the need for treatment in the long-term. It feels like I'm giving up control of my life – and that is one of my most terrible fears.'

Colm's feelings are very common. Taking any treatment, even one that is effective and safe, is a challenge for many people. The reluctance to take treatment is a complex phenomenon. It seems ironic that the recovery from a disorder that is about control requires this apparent handover of autonomy. In reality, taking treatment should not represent a loss of self-control. Taking treatment delivers a recovery that sets people free from the trap of the disorder. The decision to take treatment is the first step in an authentic journey to personal independence through mental recovery. The person who decides to take effective treatment and who recovers is in charge of their life for the first time since their disorder began.

Whereas many of us are prepared to take treatments for raised blood pressure, high cholesterol, diabetes or other medical conditions, we are less willing to take medication for mental problems. This is especially so if the treatment is prolonged. There are many factors explaining this ambivalent position, but for Colm his perceived loss of control was the major stumbling block.

We discussed the issue at length. In the end, it was Colm's decision to persist with the recovery plan.

'This time, I think I will stick with it. From now on I hope to be well – I believe I can be. I'm learning that I am only human and some things are just out of my control. And maybe that is just as well!'

In time we agreed a recovery plan that combined psychotherapy, lifestyle change and prescribed medication. I assured Colm that a care plan such as this could maintain recovery for even the most complex depressions.

Colm has remained well for over two years now. He is considering remaining on his current treatment indefinitely. He had this to say: 'If a doctor was to tell me that I have cancer, I would take the treatment. And I wouldn't think twice about it. I am going to work on getting to that point with my mental health too. I feel lucky, actually. I have the option of remaining well.'

Delight in Disorder

A sweet disorder in the dress
Kindles in clothes a wantonness;
A lawn about the shoulders thrown
Into a fine distraction;
An erring lace, which here and there
Inthralls the crimson stomacher;
A cuff neglectful, and thereby
Ribands to flow confusedly;
A winning wave, deserving note,
In the tempestuous petticoat;
A careless shoe-string, in whose tie
I see a wild civility;
Do more bewitch me, than when art
Is too precise in every part.

~

ROBERT HERRICK

Brian

For some years I used to travel to work in St Patrick's by train. In the morning I would take the forty-minute trip to Heuston Station and sit and read before coming to work, glad for the time to get myself ready for the day ahead.

One day at the park-and-ride facility, I stood waiting for my train when an expensive-looking sports car pulled up and parked nearby. The sports car was pale blue and it had leather seats. As I took a second glance, the driver of the car got out and walked towards me. As he approached, I said, somewhat clumsily: 'It's a lovely car.' He smiled at me and we got on the train.

The train wasn't full, but somehow myself and the driver of the sports car found ourselves in the same carriage, sitting opposite each other. As the train pulled away, he spoke.

'My name is Brian. How are you? Thanks for the compliment on the car. It's nice, isn't it?'

'Yes,' I said, 'it's beautiful.'

'It's Italian,' he continued. 'There are only three of them in Ireland. I have it for nearly a year now.'

I smiled and agreed with Brian that the car was certainly a thing of beauty.

Our conversation might have petered out at this point, but Brian seemed eager to talk. 'You know, I love that car – but I get no real fun out of it. I should probably leave it in the garage at home because I keep worrying that someone will take it from me. That's why I don't take it into town anymore. It's just too risky.'

'Well,' I said, 'it might be safer to leave it here then, I suppose.'

Brian continued: 'Oh, I don't know. This way is no better really.

I get the train into work so that I can leave the car here during the day – but sure, it's still on my mind all the time. I keep thinking that somebody is going to steal it. I always want to be checking it to see that it's still ok.'

Brian was cheerful but clearly found this situation distressing. 'Actually, I've recently started coming back out here to check on it during the day. I can't say anything to my boss; I just have to find ways of getting out here. I was wound up about it for some reason last Tuesday. I made three journeys out here during the day just to be certain that it hadn't been stolen. I was barely back in the office from one trip when I'd have to head back out again.'

Brian was keen to talk more about his problems. He said he was relieved to be able to share his anxiety with a total stranger. We talked freely for the rest of the journey and he shared with me many details of his life and of the stresses and worries he was experiencing. Disabling anxiety was a feature in nearly every aspect of his life and it was not just focused on his car.[1]

Most people with anxiety such as Brian's carry on without any help for years and years, truly living lives of 'quiet desperation'. When people do seek help, it is usually only in a crisis and often only after years of delay. The average duration between symptom onset of an anxiety or mood disorder and seeking professional help is about ten years.

It wasn't clear whether Brian knew that I was a psychiatrist – he didn't suggest to me that he did – but he was describing disabling worries in most areas of his life and he was clearly ill at ease. At this stage, the significance of his anxiety about his fine motorcar appeared less substantial. This worry seemed to be only one element of a much broader sense of pervasive apprehension.

I was hesitant about advising him. After all, he was a stranger and our meeting was a chance encounter. Global anxiety such as his is very common and if people in this distress seek help it is best to talk to a GP. Perhaps others would tell him to just get rid of the car, but that would not be a satisfactory response to his problem. Equally, it would have been cruel to suggest to him that he should just learn to live with the risk that it could be stolen. Then Brian said something very interesting.

'The car doesn't actually mean a whole lot to me. It's just the idea of having it stolen. I hate that feeling of not being able to protect yourself from that stuff. I mean, anything can happen. And if I can't stop stuff like that from happening, who knows where it all could end?'

I wasn't really sure what to say to Brian, but I wanted to help him so I said: 'You really should talk to someone about your anxiety – a GP or a counsellor or a very close friend who could help you. Real help is effective and you would be much more at ease if you did something about the fears you are living with.'

Brian took no offence. I have no idea whether he ever went to see his GP. A few minutes later, our train pulled into Heuston Station and we parted ways, wishing each other a good day. We have not seen each other since.

The Mower

The mower stalled, twice; kneeling, I found
A hedgehog jammed up against the blades,
Killed. It had been in the long grass.

I had seen it before, and even fed it, once.
Now I had mauled its unobtrusive world
Unmendably. Burial was no help:

Next morning I got up and it did not.
The first day after a death, the new absence
Is always the same; we should be careful

Of each other, we should be kind
While there is still time.

～

PHILIP LARKIN

Alex

Alex is a university lecturer. He asked his GP to refer him since 'he needed some help to finish his PhD', but when I saw him he complained of anxiety and a compulsive need to check everything. When he came one morning into my room, the most striking thing about him was his obvious sadness. He looked downcast and preoccupied, as though he was carrying out some mental ritual even as we spoke.

Alex is a slight young man and that first day he was wearing a clean check shirt, a sweater and new blue jeans. As we spoke he sat upon his hands, speaking softly, looking downwards towards the floor. 'The thing is this. I am writing my PhD and I just can't finish it. I cannot stop rewriting the damn chapters.'

Alex described his day. No moment was free from worry. He rose early, regardless of the fact that this was disturbing his girlfriend's sleep. Alex began each day with rituals of checking and rechecking. For him, it was imperative that the house was locked and then unlocked in a certain order each day. Each morning, he checked that the knobs on the cooker were all turned to the 'off' position; he checked that all of the doors in their small apartment were locked; and then he unlocked them in a certain order, ready for the new day. Initially, this checking behaviour seemed to relieve him of his distress but that was no longer the case.

'I used to get relief from doing these things. I don't know why. There's a feeling that if I check all these things correctly, then nothing bad can happen. I know that sounds like superstitious nonsense to most people – but what if my doing these things prevents really bad things from happening? Okay, I'm probably not stopping plane crashes or hurricanes or anything but there's something very appealing about the checking.

'I spend most of my day making sure that everything is in its place. I have my rituals, I suppose. I like being busy all the time. And in fairness, I usually get a lot done and I'm good at my work. There shouldn't be any problem with finishing my thesis. The problem is in the writing: it has to be just right. I can tell that my thesis supervisor is getting frustrated now. He's not able to get me to finish the work.'

Alex told me about his girlfriend, Julie. 'We've been together five years now. We've no kids. Things are pretty good but Julie is finding it annoying that I'm not getting this thesis done.'

Then Alex said something that was hard to put in context. 'There's something you should know about Julie: she's a stunning-looking girl. You should see her.'

Why had Alex chosen to say this about his partner? Was it a way to be charming? Was he trying to boast? I wasn't sure what was happening, but I decided to let it go. Better to say nothing and just listen and try to understand. Our session came to a close and Alex agreed to see me again.

As soon as Alex sat down at our next session, he immediately returned to the subject of his girlfriend.

'I was telling you that my girlfriend, Julie, is very beautiful. Well, I wasn't lying – she is. Something I noticed about her from the very start was that she made a big effort with her appearance. I love that. I like to see people looking the best that they possibly can. She's very pretty. I sometimes think that she's naturally so pretty that she's totally out of my league... I actually brought her with me today because I'd like you to see her.'

What had Alex hoped to achieve by bringing Julie to see me? Without giving any particular explanation, he insisted that I see her. I encouraged him to go to the waiting area and to invite her in, but

Alex replied: 'No. I want *you* to get her. I want you to bring her in. I guarantee that you'll be able to pick her out from the waiting area.'

Alex's behaviour seemed very odd. But, as before, it seemed best to go along with him and to say nothing. It was clear that Alex was controlling me and so I wondered what it must be like for Julie to live with him. I thought it would be a good idea to find out more about their relationship.

I went to the waiting area, where a number of people were sitting. Some were reading magazines while others listening to the radio. I noticed a very glamorous young woman with black hair and pale skin. She was wearing a tailored suit and high-heeled shoes. 'You must be Julie,' I said.

Once we were back in my room, Alex spoke more easily. However, Julie remained cautious and reticent as Alex described his anxiety and his many practical difficulties. He spoke about his procrastination and his need for control. I asked Julie whether she was happy to be hearing all of this.

'I don't really mind. I have come here because Alex asked me. I have become familiar with his demands over the years. It's nothing new. I'll be blunt. There is something you must understand about our relationship. There is nothing strange or unusual going on between us. There is a lot of tension sometimes but we do take care of each other. It's just that Alex checks everything. Alex checks light bulbs. Alex checks the locks. Alex checks the cooker. So it is hardly surprising that Alex checks me.'

The effect of obsessive-compulsive disorder (OCD) on human feeling and relationships is profound. It can be very painful for those witnessing OCD to see themselves relegated to the status of an obstacle impeding the demands of ritual control. Compassionate human feeling is hard to sustain when a relationship is reduced to a ritual and a human being to an obstacle in the way of order.

Julie was forthcoming: 'I think Alex has major control issues. He's very demanding. He checks objects and he checks people too.

I sometimes think he sees human beings as things that are just getting in the way of his obsessions. I know he can't help it in some ways. And I'm to blame for going along with lots of these things too. I've been thinking it over a lot recently and I realise that I've been happy that he sees me as this "perfect object".'

Alex and Julie both stated during this session that they were committed to each other but that they wanted their situation to change. They felt that the issue of Alex's thesis was bringing other issues to light for them. Without knowing it, both of them had been living lives dominated by Alex's need to meet the demands of his obsessive and compulsive character. Alex had demanded more and more control until none was available. He did not need help with the completion of his thesis. Instead, he needed to work with a cognitive behavioural therapist to overcome the trap of the obsessive life that he, and Julie, had been living.

Julie spoke about her frustrations. 'Part of me likes being on a pedestal. But then, sometimes I just want to wear what I want to wear. I just want to chill. I'm going to have to learn how to do that and Alex is going to have to learn how to live with that too.'

Our session ended on the agreement that Alex and Julie would engage in therapy together. The road ahead would be difficult for both of them. The drug of compulsive reassurance is hard to abandon for those that seek it and for those that give it. Behaviour that is controlling is hard to change, but real recovery requires that valued human relationships be given priority over the demands of private anxiety. The humdrum agenda of OCD can obscure the human feeling that exists between people caught in its wake.

—

Two years passed before Alex and Julie returned to my room. They were no longer in therapy and a new crisis had arisen quite suddenly. Throughout his recovery, Alex had been struggling to completely eliminate his need to check for contamination. Although he had reduced his checking rituals during the day, he had continued to wash his hands in a compulsive fashion each night before going to bed.

Julie had tolerated this persistent use of disinfectants late at night. She turned a blind eye to the fact that each evening, Alex would go to the utility room adjacent to their kitchen and wash his hands in disinfectant. This distressed Julie but she said little about it. The smell of the disinfectant was one thing she found difficult to bear at night but she acknowledged the progress Alex had made and the fact that he had limited his cleaning rituals to this apparently isolated nocturnal behaviour. Overall, she felt that Alex had been doing better.

So why had they come back now?

Julie explained that Alex had become acutely distressed one evening a fortnight previously and he had suddenly begun to scream and shout. The precipitant for his outburst was the fact that it was bedtime and he couldn't find his disinfectant. Julie had tidied the utility room and, without intending to upset him, she had moved the disinfectant from Alex's appointed place. When Alex went to do his usual cleaning ritual he could not find the means. He became acutely distressed, and for him this distress was too hard to contain. He screamed and he began to bang his head against the side of the kitchen door. Julie looked on, shocked and powerless, very frightened for him and equally distressed for herself.

Alex said little about this incident, while Julie spoke directly to me. 'You always said that I should not give in to his OCD, but this was a crisis and I had no choice but to do what he wanted. You said previously that the best thing in these circumstances is to refuse to co-operate with the demands of the OCD – but what was I supposed to do?

'I had to search for the disinfectant and try to give in to him. He was injuring himself. It got worse after that and he started insisting that I also wash with disinfectant and that we would have to have the house fumigated. The whole episode took hours to calm down. What could I have done? I did what you told me and look at what happened... What would you have done?'

Julie was right. I had advised them that it is better not to collude with the demands of OCD. And yet, faced with Alex's outburst, Julie was placed in an impossible situation where anyone would have acceded to the OCD demands just as Julie had done. She had behaved perfectly reasonably. When I gave this reassuring response I was shocked by Julie's angry reaction.

'How can you sit there now and give me advice about managing Alex's OCD that is so contradictory to what you said earlier? I have been worried sick because, contrary to your advice, I gave in to his demands. Your advice made me feel like a total failure! And now you say that what I did that night is all okay. If that wasn't bad enough, because of you I have been worried sick about his potential for relapse. And I've been expecting the absolute worst, because I believed that I had made things worse.'

What was there to say? Julie saw my advice as unsatisfactory and unrelated to the real world. She told me my response was 'facile'. I told them both that I was very sorry. It was not just that I had fallen into the trap of giving advice. I had not made it clear that real life requires flexibility and contains a degree of uncertainty.

Julie's response to the crisis in their kitchen had been the right one and I did not want either of them to be in any doubt about that. As adults, we have autonomy and we can make choices. It was no good that Alex continued to feel compelled by the demands of his OCD and now Julie felt equally compelled by the demands of my advice. Recovery should be liberating and a good recovery plan works because it relies upon the people in recovery to do what is best for them.

Alex and Julie decided to go back to therapy for a while. In therapy, they discussed their mutual obsessive behaviour more fully and examined the ways in which OCD thinking and behaviour was affecting them both. Once again they agreed that the logic of obsessive-compulsive anxiety is false, since the demands of OCD always start from a false premise: the obsessive insistence that any uncertainty is unacceptable.

Alex's ritual washing of his hands using disinfectant is a compulsive ritual and, like all of Alex's compulsions, it was based upon a house of cards. In order to manage the recent crisis, Julie had to compromise. Certainly, nothing would have been served by prolonging Alex's aggressive behaviour on that occasion. Julie was right when she saw that Alex's behaviour was unacceptable and that she had little choice but to go along with him at that stage. However, she also saw that appeasing his OCD had brought about an increase in his rituals and increased his reassurance-seeking. Ultimately, saying no to OCD would be the only way forward for them both. But at times, saying no has to include room for adaptation.

It was also true that Alex was very ashamed of his behaviour and he reproached himself for it. In therapy, he realised that he wanted to express his gratitude to Julie for her love for him: 'Without a doubt, Julie has been the biggest reason for my recovery.'

Timing is everything. Before his crisis, Alex had taken advantage of his earlier progress to continue his ritual use of disinfectant even after the other compulsions were diminished. To put it another way, Alex had kept his compulsive behaviour as a hostage. And in the end, hostages always have to be released.

Julie had been conflicted. Her pragmatic compromise for the man she loved clashed with her desire to see the authentic way forward.

It was clear that Alex and Julie were now in this therapy together. Their recovery would be a joint achievement, an act of union, with new thinking all round.

Postscript

And some time make the time to drive out west
Into County Clare, along the Flaggy Shore,
In September or October, when the wind
And the light are working off each other
So that the ocean on one side is wild
With foam and glitter, and inland among stones
The surface of a slate-grey lake is lit
By the earthed lightning of a flock of swans,
Their feathers roughed and ruffling, white on white,
Their fully grown headstrong-looking heads
Tucked or cresting or busy underwater.
Useless to think you'll park and capture it
More thoroughly. You are neither here nor there,
A hurry through which known and strange things pass
As big soft buffetings come at the car sideways
And catch the heart off guard and blow it open.

~

SEAMUS HEANEY

Memory

Recovery from mental disorder is more likely when people engage with care. This may seem facile, but it is true. Those who engage with recovery have a much better outlook than those who do not. While some individuals seek help actively and thus take decisive steps towards learning and recovery, for other patients engagement with mental health care comes more obliquely. For them, learning begins as a result of circumstances out of their control. Whether the pretext for seeking help and engaging in recovery is conscious and intentional, by accident, in an acute crisis, or even in the context of chronic decline, the capacity to recover depends in large part on the brain's ability to change and to grow.

Much has been learned about fundamental brain processes over the past hundred years. Since Freud and his colleagues described the unconscious mechanisms of the mind, and Pavlov trained his dogs to associate feeding time with the ringing of a bell (in a learning process we now call 'conditioning'), psychologists, neurologists and psychiatrists have together been studying the process of learning, providing more and more understanding of the workings of the human brain.

In modern mental health care, these clinical neurosciences come together in teams, combining new psychological understandings with biological insights gleaned from brain imaging and molecular biological techniques. Working together in multidisciplinary teams helps everyone to understand more about how mental health works and also about why it breaks down. While we still know far too little about the detailed workings of the brain, as a result of this shared neuroscience, there is greater reason for hope that we can develop more effective ways to harness the brain's capacity for learning and recovery. One development arising from this shared scientific approach has been the confirmation that early intervention is a key to recovery.

Healthy brain function maintains human equilibrium and functional social integrity. This is true whether we are talking of motor abilities or cognitive functions or of any of the complex inter-related faculties that depend upon the intact brain. Disintegration of the relationship between thoughts and emotions, or between memories and fears, is a common hallmark of the suffering experienced by those with clinical depression and anxiety disorder. Modern psychotherapies such as cognitive behavioural therapy (CBT) and mindfulness techniques work in part by reintegrating these functions. Thus, they confirm the centrality of the brain in our ability to recover.

There has been a great deal of controversy regarding the phenomenon of recovered memory. This divisive debate came to a peak more than twenty years ago when some therapists claimed repressed or dissociated memories had to be recovered in order to allow each person to 'heal'. While some others dismissed these recollections as insignificant, the terrible truth about physical and sexual abuse in childhood has emerged distressingly over the years.

Physical and sexual abuse of children is a very large problem in our society and in many cases, disclosure does not come about unless a person is specifically asked. In Ireland the policy guidelines known as Children First have been helpful, and these guidelines do facilitate disclosure wherever there is a 'reasonable' suspicion that abuse has occurred. The recent amendment to Ireland's constitution incorporating a new article on children's rights (Article 42A) is a hopeful and positive step forward. The legislative basis for protection of children is likely to be reinforced by its successful adoption by our people.

The stories of Dorothy, Jack and Margaret illustrate the

importance of understanding the relationship between the brain, behaviour and memory in patients with depression or anxiety disorder. The ability to recollect is a key function. Clinically, we still have much to learn about how we remember. We must also learn how it is – and why it is – that we forget.

Dorothy

Dorothy is an 82-year-old retired teacher, a widow and a mother of two adult children, Ellen and Timothy. Late one evening, Dorothy was found wandering in a public car park near O'Connell Street in Dublin. Lost and utterly unaware of her place in time, she could not remember her name or recognise a single person.

The ambulance brought Dorothy to a nearby hospital from where she was admitted to a medical bed in the emergency department. Dorothy had a fever. Analysis of her urine revealed that she had an infection which had probably caused her acute confusion and precipitated her wandering from home.

The nurses began trying to identify Dorothy and, within a matter of hours, her daughter was located using details they found in Dorothy's handbag. Dorothy's daughter, Ellen, had been frantically searching for her mother for more than a day, and so she had contacted the Gardaí to report her mother missing.

Three years earlier, Dorothy's husband had died. Since then, Dorothy had been living with Ellen and her husband, and their three young children. The family welcomed Dorothy into their home as their much-loved granny. Secure in their company, Dorothy felt able to grieve for the loss of her husband, her home and her independence. Three or four times a year, Dorothy's spirits were lifted by a visit from her son, Timothy, who would travel from the us where he lived and worked.

Dorothy had been struggling to maintain her memory for facts and events, and Ellen realised that her mother's ability to function independently had been in steady decline. In recent years, Dorothy had suffered a series of small stokes, which decreased her mental reserve bit by bit. Now in the busy setting of the medical ward, Dorothy deteriorated even further. Functions she had maintained for years, things she had been able to sustain in familiar surroundings, were lost rapidly in the alien environment of the general hospital. Although no longer distressed or feverish, Dorothy quickly became mute and uncommunicative. Dorothy's family arranged to move her from the general hospital to St Patrick's, where she stayed for a time.

Ellen came to see me in my room one day and she explained that she was keen to take her mother home as soon as possible.

'I have discussed it at home and with my brother, Timothy, in the States. We all know it's going to be challenging, but we really want to try to care for Mum at home in my house.'

After a brief stay at St Patrick's, Dorothy's clinical team recommended a trial of discharge, with support from Dorothy's GP and a carer provided by an agency dedicated to care of the elderly in a home setting. Ellen and her family were apprehensive but determined. 'We really want to have Mum with us for as long as we can. I know that's what she would like us to do.'

Dorothy's birthday would be a few days after her return home, so Ellen was planning a family party. 'It'll be really nice for the children. They've missed having Granny in the house. This way, we get to celebrate her birthday and her return home to us. And the big event is that Timothy's coming home from the States. He's bringing his partner and their two kids. It'll be really sweet. We've had great parties over the years, so it'll be just like old times.'

Timothy arrived safely with his family and settled in to Ellen's home for a few days. However, it was clear that Dorothy didn't recognise him, his partner or their children. Timothy soon learned from Ellen that Dorothy had not really connected with anyone since her return home. The distress that Ellen and Timothy felt was visceral.

The day of the party arrived and there was a flurry of activity. The children made cards, Timothy set the tables, Ellen baked a cake – everybody was given something to do.

As the evening drew in, guests started to arrive. All the old friends and neighbours came to see Dorothy, but she seemed to recognise nobody. She sat in a chair in the kitchen, mute and unaware. When friends greeted her, she responded with a vacant smile. There was nothing that could be done.

Dorothy remained for some time in the kitchen. Then, without invitation or prompting, she stood up. She moved towards the piano in the living room. She sat down and began to play. Throughout her life, Dorothy had been an enthusiastic piano player. 'The West's Awake' was one of her favourite pieces. She had played that tune at many parties. Now, seemingly detached, she played it once again. She didn't stumble or make any error. The guests looked on, spellbound.

Dorothy's knowledge of faces, facts and events had almost completely disappeared. It seemed that her knowledge of how to play the piano had been preserved, despite her amnesia for everything else. In order to understand Dorothy's brain decline, it is helpful to know that memories can be divided into distinct groups, which map onto separate brain processes and distinct brain circuits. Nobel laureate Professor Eric Kandel teaches us that one form of memory is concerned with Knowing How (knowledge of motor skills) while another form of memory is concerned with Knowing That (knowledge of facts and events). Knowing how to do things is expressed through performance and does not require conscious recollection of past data. This 'how to do' memory involves specific motor pathways deep in the brain.

In truth, the organ that we call 'the brain' includes many 'organs'. These include structures in the outer cortex, along with deep brain structures such as the cerebellum, the amygdala and the basal ganglia. Memory for how to do things integrates behaviours such as the performance of ordinary motor habits and long-learned motor skills such as touch-typing, playing tennis or playing a musical instrument. These are very similar to processes amenable to classical conditioning, which Pavlov studied over a hundred years ago.

In Dorothy's dementia, her memory loss had been initially the loss of Knowing That (knowledge of facts and events).[1] This form of memory loss involves the loss of conscious focused cortical attention. Dorothy had lost functions dependent on the outer area of her brain, the cerebral cortex and in particular the medial temporal cortical system and the hippocampus.

But Dorothy's memory of how to play the piano depended on the function of deeper structures in her brain, which had not yet entirely declined. Without a functioning temporal cortical system, she could not recollect facts or events. Nevertheless, through circumstances out of her control, Dorothy revealed an important lesson. Interrelated brain functions are distinct and they decline at different rates. Dorothy's memory for Knowing That had been lost, but her memory for Knowing How had been preserved – at least for a time.

In caring for Dorothy, we would focus on her dignity and human rights. We would prioritise her preserved abilities so that she might enjoy as many of these qualities as possible, and for as long as possible.

Ellen came to see me in my room a few days after Dorothy's birthday party. 'You'd have to have been there to see it and hear it. It really was the strangest thing. I was distressed at first, but there was something about the music. I don't know. We just watched it all unfold. Really, these are the good moments – for all of us involved. We have to enjoy them while we can.'

Piano

Softly, in the dusk, a woman is singing to me;
Taking me back down the vista of years, till I see
A child sitting under the piano, in the boom of the tingling strings
And pressing the small, poised feet of a mother who smiles as she sings.

In spite of myself, the insidious mastery of song
Betrays me back, till the heart of me weeps to belong
To the old Sunday evenings at home, with winter outside
And hymns in the cosy parlour, the tinkling piano our guide.

So now it is vain for the singer to burst into clamour
With the great black piano appassionato. The glamour
Of childish days is upon me, my manhood is cast
Down in the flood of remembrance, I weep like a child for the past.

∾

D.H. LAWRENCE

Jack

J ack is a 50-year-old man who came seeking help for his low mood. Jack's GP referred him because of Jack's symptoms of deep melancholy and despair over many months. Jack's sadness was so severe that he had repeatedly attempted suicide, with many hospitalisations and a number of failed trials with antidepressants. Jack had a recurrent depressive disorder.[1] This is a form of disordered mood that can occur despite the best efforts of the patient and regardless of the treatment chosen.

Jack told me about himself. 'I've been living with my partner for five years now. We're hard workers. We're in computer software. We started in boom times but we're still doing grand in the recession. It's not so bad that way. I get a lot from work. I'm better when I'm busy. Hate being idle. If I'm not busy, the demons come out.'

When describing life at home, Jack said: 'I know I've a good partner. At the same time, I know I can be a real bastard to live with. We've had our rows. There was never any violence or anything. But there were times when I said rotten stuff. Really rotten stuff. I feel guilty about that. We haven't rowed for a long time now. I'm just depressed and I can't shake it.'

The problem for Jack was not conspicuously related to memory, but in talking about his life it gradually became clear that Jack had very few recollections of his childhood. He certainly had no happy ones.

'My father was rough, so I don't dwell on childhood. I don't have that many memories – probably better off. I'd say I've completely forgotten lots of things that happened. I do remember my father being useless, though. He was useless and very angry. He beat me so badly on my thirteenth birthday that I actually broke down. I was weeping and begging him to stop. And he just didn't. From then on, I was done with him. I swore that day that I would never cry over him again. I didn't even cry the day they buried him.'

In understanding Jack's story, we have to consider the processes underlying suppression of recollection. It is understood that memory for Knowing That (memory for facts and events) includes two subtypes of memory processes: the first is concerned with general knowledge about the data (semantic memory) but the second recalls the context and significance of events (episodic memory).

On reflection, Jack agreed that it would not be true to say that he had completely forgotten lots of things. 'No, I haven't forgotten my childhood, but I don't have many memories of it. I don't dwell on that stuff. I'm more interested in getting out of this depression.'

Jack had never connected his traumatic experiences in childhood with his recurrent depression or his anger. Jack's memory failure was not a loss of semantic memory. Indeed he had never entirely forgotten these things. Jack's episodic memory had been suppressed but not entirely lost. There many facts associated with the painful context of his childhood that were unbearable and so, in order to survive, he had suppressed them. In effect, he had suppressed the significance of these events in order to avoid the pain associated with them. Jack had depression in the context of a state of extreme emotional self-control. His mental self-defence was so intense, that his capacity for joy had been controlled and almost completely extinguished. His struggle for control consumed almost all of his emotional energy and extinguished almost all of his hope.

Jack needed to see his own short temper and his flashes of anger as a reaction to this suppression. If he saw his anger as a disproportionate response to his trauma and to his defences, it could help him to understand his behaviour and move on from his punitive self-reproach. If Newton's laws of physics applied to mental health, this would mean that to every emotional action there would be an equal and opposite emotional reaction. For Jack, suppressing his anger in one location inevitably caused it to appear somewhere else. The more he suppressed his emotional life the more it would emerge elsewhere in his experience. Jack agreed to ponder this.

As we talked over the coming weeks, Jack began to acknowledge that his real pain was in his past. 'Yeah, there was a lot of pain there for me. And I was just a kid. Looking at it now, there was a lot of pain. It's weird because it's in the past. So it's over, but it's not.'

It was clear that Jack's recovery would not be an easy or a rapid process. However, in one way, it was helpful to address his memory difficulty, to contextualise his suffering, so that he could begin to feel again and so to recover once more. He agreed to enter a period of longer-term psychotherapy with one of our clinical psychologists.

With the help of his partner, Jack has been on a psychotherapeutic journey for some time now. It has been an extended expedition of hope. Over time in psychotherapy, each element of Jack's personal regrowth represented a spark of new learning and the discovery of a new interpersonal insight. As Jack has recovered, he has stored in his consciousness each authentic new meaning, in emotional and cognitive places that were previously bleak and where only painful experiences had been stored.

Most memories of childhood trauma have never been forgotten, even if (as in Jack's case) their emotional context has been blunted and their eventual disclosure delayed. The debate about recovered memory should not be used to deny justice to victims of abuse. The abuse of children is a crime. Memories of abuse may be undisclosed for many years.

Jack's recollection was valid and accurate, but his detachment from its context and its pain had suffocated his emotional life and hindered his recovery. In therapy, Jack has learned to rediscover his feelings, the integrity of his memories and the coherence of the emotions connected to them. Today he is less depressed. With this recovery, his mind functions more fully as the conscious arbiter of his feelings and of his recollections.

Recently we spoke in my room. Jack said: 'I think I'm getting to know my own mind better, now that I'm looking at things. Do you know that phrase? "Whatever you say, say nothing." That could've been my motto before. I'm getting over that idea, though. I'm talking more – and not just with a shrink, by the way! No – I'm definitely talking more at home too. Because time just seemed to go by before. Years go by. Stuff gets jammed up and then it's too much. Yeah… I'm getting there. I'm probably looking back on things differently now.'

My Papa's Waltz

The whiskey on your breath
Could make a small boy dizzy;
But I hung on like death:
Such waltzing was not easy.

We romped until the pans
Slid from the kitchen shelf;
My mother's countenance
Could not unfrown itself.

The hand that held my wrist
Was battered on one knuckle;
At every step you missed
My right ear scraped a buckle.

You beat time on my head
With a palm caked hard by dirt,
Then waltzed me off to bed
Still clinging to your shirt.

~

THEODORE ROETHKE

Margaret

If events had not taken the course they did, Margaret might never have come to see a psychiatrist.

The day began for Margaret like so many other days. She was under pressure and was rushing to take a taxi. She recalled the cleanliness of the taxi and the strong smell of lavender that came from an air freshener dangling from the driver's rear view mirror. She remembered very little else about the dreadful road traffic accident that followed, except for the extremely loud noise of the collision and the shock of the impact, which was so severe that she began to throw up over the seat. The sour taste of vomit spilling from her stomach filled the back of her throat and was embedded in her memory.

What happened immediately afterwards piled more trauma on top of trauma. With a struggle, Margaret managed to undo her seat belt and escaped out of the passenger door and onto the road. Unfortunately, as she did so, Margaret was struck for a second time – this time by the side of an oncoming vehicle and she was thrown back onto the central reservation of the dual carriage way.

Margaret described her story with no awareness of her bravery or her bewilderment. Amazingly, she had made a full physical recovery so that, apparently, she was able to go back to work within a few months.

Initially, Margaret's suffering involved only minor bruising and a few broken bones. She had no evidence of brain damage: her scans were all normal. But some months later, Margaret began to experience panic attacks. Despite her best efforts, she suffered from sudden bursts of extreme anxiety of such high intensity that with each crescendo of terror she thought she was going to die. These panic episodes were typically precipitated by loud noises or by the smell of strong perfumes or by the nauseating taste of vomit in the back of her throat.

Margaret described the story of her accident fluently but quietly. She blamed herself for her responses. She had been doing everything in her power to adapt to her distress, but she had begun to avoid going out, so as to spare herself the experience of panic attacks. Prompted by the slightest of reminders, she experienced vivid intrusive memories by day and distressing horrific nightmares by night. These vivid and intrusive recollections of an event are sometimes called flashbacks and they intruded upon Margaret's mind despite her best efforts to resist them. These unwanted tormentors left Margaret in a state of constant vigilance and invariably without a full night's sleep. As Margaret described her story, it was clear that she met diagnostic criteria for post-traumatic stress disorder (PTSD).[1]

Each day Margaret relived the dreadful intensity of her initial experience in the form of intrusive memories. Her memory disturbance was exacerbated not only by re-experiencing of the original horrific event but also by further traumas and more day-to-day losses of a lesser magnitude. In our conversations, she described multiple renewed prompts for her distress. Margaret was uncontrollably re-experiencing the original trauma and reliving it in the present. Objectively, the trauma was over but for Margaret it did not feel like that: 'It just keeps happening again and again, over and over in my mind and in my body.'

Margaret's mind was filled with evocative distressing sounds, smells and tastes. The brain circuits for these senses (smell, taste and sound) are located close to each other in the cortex, the temporal lobe, the amygdala and the hippocampus. The work of integrating experience and emotion with memory and function is done in these highly interconnected areas of the brain. The diffuse systems and regions integrating these very human functions in Margaret's brain were in overdrive, and so she looked for help.

Part of Margaret's difficulty was her disbelief at what had happened to her. As she strove unsuccessfully to put the thoughts and images of her accident out of her head, she felt emotionally numb. 'I know I am very lucky to be alive but I cannot understand why this should have happened to me in the first place. None of it makes any sense.'

Margaret spoke of her other difficulties. 'You know, I haven't had an easy life so far. I had a very difficult childhood and I haven't had an easy time of it since then either. Mam died when I was small. It was awful.

'Things have been really tough in recent years. My partner walked out on me and I've been raising our three children by myself. They're in school, so I go out to work – but it's not an easy situation.

'I feel very isolated and very alone at times since the separation. And that hasn't been clear-cut, either: we're still in legal battles over different things.

'I do have family. My older sister is good to me. She always has been. She was great when Mam died. She looked after me. She was really good after the separation too – really kind to the kids. She's always saying I should try to get out more. To be honest, it's hard to listen to her at times. I mean, it's all well and good saying I should try to start over. But I'm thinking: the life I've already had has been hard enough, so why would I go out looking for a new one?'

Was Margaret suffering from depression? She had multiple depressive and anxious symptoms.

'My sleep is totally gone, so I've no energy. I don't even have the will to eat a lot of the time. I can't remember the last time I looked forward to anything. I'm just existing. And I'm existing for the kids – because they need me. I think I'm totally traumatised.

'Then I wonder what is the use of being here? Why come here just to get a label? Will it make any difference if I say that I'm depressed or I'm traumatised? What can that do? Is a label going to find me a partner who will stick with me? Will a label roll back time? Will it bring back my mother? Will it help me to raise the kids? Will it stop the accident going around and around my head every single day? I just think I'm better off forgetting as much of it as possible.'

How should we respond to Margaret's distress? Simple reassurance is all very well, but there is no evidence that soft words, however sincere, are effective therapy. Of course kindness must be the therapeutic starting point, but Margaret made it clear that she had come for professional help for her traumatic symptoms. She was finding it hard to cope day-to-day.

'I'm finding it very difficult to sleep. Work is becoming a struggle. I feel like it's all becoming a nightmare. I need help. I am no longer the mistress of my own mind.'

Somehow we had to establish the therapeutic facts. Recovery is possible. In fact, the most likely outcome after any trauma is recovery. Margaret needed help to empower her journey towards that freedom. The treatment plan could help to give her back the mastery of her mind and the control of her life.

Margaret's recovery would not be a fiction. It would not require magic or the achievement of the impossible. Recovery does not depend on bringing back the dead or dragging an estranged husband from another relationship. With Margaret's trust and with her recovery as the goal, we set about trying to find an authentic intervention.

The understanding of Margaret's clinical symptoms has come a long way in the past thirty years. When considering Margaret's symptoms, it was helpful to her to hear just how far this has come. In the past, people with depression were erroneously divided into two groups. The first group were believed to have features of depression in response to life's difficult circumstances. This was so-called 'reactive depression'. The reactive depression was seen as being secondary to events, with a clear precipitating cause. The patient's experience of sadness and joylessness was supposed to respond to the resolution of these precipitants.

Reactive depression was thought to be quite distinct from 'endogenous depression', in which no clear precipitant was objectively evident. The features of endogenous depression were more likely to involve severe sleep disturbance, marked weight loss, impaired facility for thinking and even irrational or delusional thoughts. Whereas reactive depression had a presumed personal, psychological or social management, endogenous depression generally required a chemical treatment.

Almost nothing about this 'reactive/endogenous' classification turned out to be correct or true. The research evidence has disproved it and confirmed that binary ideological thinking does not help to deepen our understanding of problems such as Margaret's. The reactive/endogenous classification has been abandoned in mental health care for very good reasons. Firstly, the stress (or lack of stress) precipitating mental disorder does not predict its course or treatment. Whether there is a reaction of some kind, the patient's subjective understanding does not benefit from objective condescension by the therapist. Who is to say which stress is justified or significant? One man's loss may be insignificant to another. Universally, depression is loss enough to warrant acknowledgement and respect.

Recovery planning for mental distress is effective regardless of the source of the trauma. It is not necessary or practicable to expect the precipitants of depression to be resolved or to base treatment on the removal of any causal event. Modern treatm⌐ for depression and anxiety integrates real experiences (or lac⌐ with authentic interventions. The result should be plan which is pragmatic and based on proven evi⌐ outcome for Margaret would be to foster her en⌐ this could lead to measurable personal eviden⌐

Margaret's depression occurred in a social context of objective stress, trauma and great personal loss. In her recovery journey, we acknowledged all of this. Her clinical depression needed a response that was psychological, social and biological. There is no useful ideological division between therapeutic responses to human suffering. In practice, with each patient the treatment plan needs to be individualised and each treatment plan must put the rights and needs of the patient first. Margaret needed treatment that included intervention based on evidence of proven effectiveness. Her recovery plan also needed to be holistic and informed by social, psychological and biological research.

The seminal sociological research work of Brown and Harris compellingly demonstrated the relationship between life events, chronic social stress and depression. In 1978 Brown and Harris published their studies on depressed women in inner city London, in which the researchers identified several factors that increased the risk of developing depression after life events. These risk factors in the depressed women included: a lack of a confiding adult relationship; unemployment; and having three or more children under the age of 14 at home. The crucial background variable in the clinical depression experienced by these women after major stress was the loss of their own mother, particularly when this bereavement was premature and occurred before they reached the age of 11.

It was clear that Margaret had suffered many losses in her life, but she dismissed each of them as irrelevant to her current distress. The death of her mother effectively ended her childhood, and the recent loss of her husband brought to an end her hopes for resolved family life as she might have imagined it. The trauma of her road traffic accident was a major stress; it limited her independence as a consequence of her avoidance and her newfound hypervigilance and intrusive thoughts. Margaret had seen no connection between these earlier losses and her current state of distress. As far as she was concerned, these issues were surely irrelevant and so she had 'put them well out of her mind'.

Margaret's symptoms of depression and PTSD arose from more than her recent traffic accident but her recognition of this was limited. She was clinically depressed, anxious and seriously traumatised, but she was utterly unaware of the connections between her current post-traumatic state and the long-standing grief she carried with her throughout life. Neither did she see a connection between the hardship she was experiencing in her life and her current symptoms of low mood and despair.

Margaret said she wanted to be heard. Listening to her trauma could help build understanding and help her connect the strands of her painful journey. For her, life was just a series of painful losses. As she put it: 'My life is just one damn thing after another.' Perhaps she could begin to see her life in a connected way and begin a journey of real understanding to mitigate her current distress. If we could link her sadness to her losses, and her trauma to her avoidance, she could start to make sense of it all and begin what we later called her 'whole new plan for living'.

Listening to suffering is not easy, but listening is a vital part of a psychiatrist's work. For any clinical therapist it is essential to listen in a very special way. As Daniel Barenboim puts it: 'Listening is hearing with thought; just as feeling is emotion with thought.' In responding to Margaret's pain, we would need to work together to do this enhanced listening, but Margaret's persistent adherence to a serial view of her problems made it hard to build a common understanding. She repeatedly dismissed reflection on events, and so it became hard to outline a recovery plan.

'We could go over the same ground and get nowhere, doctor. I just have to face up to it. Shit happens. And in my life, it happens again and again. I wouldn't be surprised if you're sick of listening to me. I feel like everyone's sick of listening to me – apart from my sister. Maybe.'

Could Margaret reflect on her life as a constructive narrative, rather than as a series of bad episodes? In order to be therapeutic, we would have to co-operate with each other and with other members of the multidisciplinary team. Margaret would need to be willing to integrate her life experiences with the life of her mind, and to stay the course. Therapy could include cognitive behavioural therapy (CBT) with real-life exposure and homework and possibly even medication. It would not be easy but, with a recovery plan, Margaret would begin to overcome her avoidance and anxiety. By agreeing to let go of her scepticism, her melancholy could begin to melt. New enduring positive experiences could emerge from the cold.

At our later meetings, Margaret agreed to work on a plan towards her targets and her personal goals. The evidence of research in psychotherapy supports this. Recovery occurs through repeated restorative exposure combined with learning.[2] With experience the brain grows and reconnects experience to meaning, binding the senses afresh with constructive emotions, with new thoughts and new feelings, new sounds and new relationships. This reconnection is personal regrowth and it builds new understanding to deliver healing and further recovery.

Once she agreed to work on her recovery plan, Margaret began to experience a new way forward. In therapy she acknowledged the unconscious traps posed by her fear of abandonment, and she no longer dismissed these hazards as insignificant. She dedicated herself to greater understanding of her life and of her future.

'Something interesting came up in therapy. I realised that I dismiss others because that's my defence against my ultimate fear, which is that I will be dismissed myself. I'm learning a lot in therapy. I feel like I'm knitting myself back to together again. I live in real-time now. I feel like I'm present. I know I'll need support in the future, but I'm determined to stay well.'

New Every Morning

Every day is a fresh beginni
Listen my soul to the glad re
And, spite of old sorrows
And older sinning,
Troubles forecasted
And possible pain,
Take heart with the day and begin again.

∽

SUSAN COOLIDGE

Truth

Our society is in denial regarding the mental health problems of addiction and alcohol dependence. An authentic message about substance use and relaxation is not easy to find in Ireland today. Culturally it is difficult for us to regard a sober life as potentially a joyful one, as our reflex is to associate alcohol consumption with almost every life event and especially with times of celebration, fun and recreation. Look at the success of the lobby encouraging us to associate the use of alcohol with sport. Its force is so powerful that we have come to fear for the continuity of some of our most important cultural activities unless we co-operate with the consumption myth. Our society talks from time to time about the problems caused by alcohol and substance misuse, but it is the patients and families with depression, anxiety and addiction who face these challenges every day and they must wonder who is listening to them.

Alcohol addiction causes more damage to Irish society than most other mental problems combined, but we rarely consider alcohol as being one of the risk factors we need to worry about for our own mental wellbeing. Alcohol is a mood-altering substance and long-term addiction can cause irreparable damage to individuals and their families. When we 'self-medicate' with alcohol as a way of dealing with our mental distress, the problems of life do not go away. Instead, alcohol amplifies them, and brings with it new dimensions all of its own.

Eoin

Eoin is a teacher in a large national school near Dublin. His GP had been treating him for depression. After a brief improvement in mood, Eoin relapsed and become apathetic and so his GP referred him. The GP's referral letter described Eoin as a dedicated teacher, a married man and a father of two young boys. The letter noted that he had recently resigned from his role as deputy principal at his school and that there seemed to be a lot of stress at home.

When Eoin came to my room, he told me that he was ambivalent about seeing a psychiatrist. 'My wife says it is necessary and so I have agreed to go along with it. Anyway, I suppose it is possible that you might be able to help me.'

Eoin sat calmly in my room, without any obvious distress. He was alert and fluent and forthcoming, and despite his declaration of lowered mood, there was no sign that his mental function was slowed up in any way. His appearance was fine and his physique athletic.

'My mood is low, I suppose. But I'm healthy all the same. Going to the gym is a great relief to me. When I'm exercising, it lifts my mood and I sleep better. I find that strenuous exercise is much better than the tablets my doctor prescribed. I just felt deadened on the SSRIs he gave me. And worse still, my libido went right out the window. I was less anxious on them for sure, but it wasn't what I'd call living.'

Eoin spoke at ease about the problems he was having and why he had resigned as deputy principal. 'It just wasn't worth all the stress involved. I used to enjoy the teaching and I like the kids, but everything was getting on top of me. The expectations of the parents and their multiple demands were increasing all the time.'

While Eoin knew that his mood was low, he could not say he had ever felt despair or ever experienced a definite longing for death. Profound depressions invariably include some kind of death-wish at some stage. Interestingly, this was entirely absent in Eoin's presentation. He explained that as well as feeling low, he was not able to enjoy anything and he was no longer looking forward to any of his usual activities. This is a symptom known as anhedonia and, along with lowered mood, it is essential for a diagnosis of depression.

Eoin denied substantial difficulty with his concentration, despite his recent loss of motivation for work or sport.

'I don't have the same motivation at work and yes, I'm not going to football any more. But I'm not really suffering with my concentration. I get things done. I'm going to work as normal, I'm eating as normal – the routine's the same… My sleep is very poor, though. I find it hard to get off to sleep. I lie awake worrying about everything and about nothing.'

Mild depressions are often associated with difficulty getting off to sleep and this is sometimes called initial insomnia. This can be distinguished from sleep disturbance in moderate or severe depressions where middle or late insomnia is more typical, and this is sometimes called early morning wakening.[1]

Eoin had few of the features seen in a moderate or severe episode of depressive disorder. He had no panic episodes and, notwithstanding his anxiety and stress, he had never missed a day from work. He summed things up as follows.

'I can see I have been struggling with life over the past six months. Perhaps it is just the stress of work that is getting me down. The deputy job was stressful, so I had no choice but to resign.'

As with any mental disorder, a clinical diagnosis of depression requires evidence to confirm that problems are associated with substantial impairment in daily functioning: personal, social or occupational. In response to his difficulties, Eoin had resigned a senior position but he was still functioning in most other areas of his life relatively well – or so it first seemed.

'We have no big financial problems. Even though borrowing money would have been easy in the boom years, we didn't do that. Marion, my wife, would never have allowed me to stray into debt. We are coping with the wage cutbacks and the levies, like everyone else in Ireland. We have been a bit more careful with our spending this past year or so, but we have no real debts. We've both kept our jobs. Thankfully, we have no real financial problems.'

Eoin was describing symptoms of distress that fell some way short of a diagnosis of depressive disorder, even a mild depressive episode.[2] Regarding treatment, however, Eoin had a fair point. There is convincing evidence that exercise and lifestyle changes can be as effective for lowered mood as medication or psychotherapy, and this is so especially for mild depressive disorders. Eoin resisted questions about his lifestyle. He dismissed any deeper enquiry about his habits. 'Look, I am a man of moderation in most things. I don't smoke, even if I do like my pint.'

Once our discussion moved to the subject of his marriage and family, Eoin surprised me.

'I should tell you that my wife is having an affair with one of her colleagues. They are both teachers in the same school and I think she has been with him for quite a few years, actually. I have suspected the affair for at least two or three years. Our youngest boy is eight years old, so it could be going on for even longer. I just cannot be sure about the timing. She denies it all whenever I confront her.

'I love Marion but I hate this situation. And I'm going to get her to admit what she's done. I haven't decided how I'll handle *him*. I may not be able to have him removed from his job, but I ca[n] life very uncomfortable for them both. I don't think th management would be too happy to hear about the situation.'

Eoin's anger and his sense of righteousness were striking.

'Of *course* she denies it! What else would she do? I've seen the way she looks at him, though. I've confronted her. I know she's sleeping with him. I've told her. I've had my suspicions for some time now and we've had rows about it. I am quite sure that she came very close to admitting it to me recently.'

What did Eoin mean by 'confronting' Marion? Eoin minimised their rows at first but then he admitted that he had been pursuing Marion about the issue.

'We discuss it every week. Sometimes we'll talk about nothing else through a whole weekend. Yes, she does get upset that I'm suspicious of her. Of course she denies it all.

'I thought about hiring a private detective to have her followed but so far I have decided against it. They would find nothing because they would have to get into her school and get pictures of her comings and goings and it could be very messy.

'I followed her recently. I had to find the proof of what I knew. I followed her and she went back into the school after the school day had ended. That was proof enough for me. There could be no other reason for her going back except to meet with him.'

Eoin had no sightings or evidence. 'No, I haven't actually seen them together. It is only a matter of time, though. She will have to admit it.'

Eoin denied that he had ever threatened his wife and he vehemently d͟e͟n͟i͟e͟d that he had ever been violent. 'I have never been phy͟s͟i͟c͟a͟l͟ ͟ and I never would be.'

ce is a very common hidden problem in Ireland derestimate it. Many people conceal domestic shame associated with the problem, as well h revealing it. At the extreme end, jealousy easons given by men who go on to murder mestic violence are very real.

Eoin seemed convinced of Marion's infidelity. 'How can I be sure? But sure it's obvious to anyone who's paying attention! You can tell from her clothes and from the perfume she wears. She only wears them for him. I've noticed the way she dresses. And I've checked her belongings for any signs of intimacy.'

Clinically, Eoin was describing a rare condition known as morbid (alcoholic) jealousy or the Othello syndrome.[3] Confidentiality has its limits and principal amongst these limits are details regarding potential harm to others. It seemed that Eoin's wife, Marion, must be under enormous pressure. Regardless of the truth of his accusations, I needed to establish whether she was safe or at risk. Since Eoin had told me that his wife encouraged him to come, it was possible she might also agree to come to my room. Hopefully he would allow me speak to her on my own. I asked him to bring Marion the very next day and to my great relief he said he would.

Marion is an impressive woman. As she spoke to me, Eoin agreed to wait outside my room. Marion described her husband and their marriage and their recent lack of sexual intimacy. Marion was more straightforward than her husband and she was very keen to be helpful.

'The first thing you need to know is that I want to keep my marriage and that I love my husband. I am not having an affair and I haven't withdrawn from Eoin, but he is a very heavy drinker and his demands for reassurance about our relationship are becoming incessant. These demands are always associated with his binges, but they used to be at the weekends only. Recently he is drinking midweek as well, and when he drinks he always gets drunk. His demands for reassurance come thick and fast once he has drink in him. I am tired of reassuring him and drunken sex is not for me.'

I asked Marion why the use of an SSRI was so unacceptable to Eoin.

'He says his libido went out the window when he was on the SSRI. But overall, he was much better when he was on medication.

Of course, he couldn't drink alcohol when he was on them. Yes, he had impotency issues when he was on the medication and I know that really got to him. He'd get frustrated and if he drank he got quite bitter. Then the questions about my fidelity would start. I'm not surprised to hear that he has denied any substance abuse, but he is addicted to alcohol. You should know that.'

There were many questions to ask about Marion's safety, but she was eager to put those concerns away.

'He has never been violent and, believe me, I am not just "standing by my man". I could not tolerate violence or threats of it – but Eoin needs help and it is clear to me that his alcohol use is really getting out of hand over the last few years. He has tried to stop and whenever he cuts alcohol out for a few months or more, our life together becomes so much better. But each time, he has returned to drinking alcohol. And each time, it's actually worse than it was before. I am worried for our boys. They love their Dad. I am just hoping that this can be helped. I don't believe that Eoin needs to get sober for me or for the boys. He needs to get sober for himself. That is the reason for all of this. His problem is that he has no regard for himself and that's the love he needs to regain. I am just hoping he can. Our kids want this as well, but he can't do it while he continues to drink in this way.'

Later on Eoin sat in my room while Marion waited outside. Eoin stared out the window. He said nothing for some time and then he spoke.

'You see? I was right. She *didn't* tell you I was a danger to her, did she? I have never been any threat. Never. Why did you have to bring her in here to tell you something that I had already told you?'

In response to this kind of challenge it would be too easy to match confrontation with more confrontation. The hopeful way forward was to make an alliance with Eoin in which we would begin to make the journey for his recovery. I thanked him for co-operating with the risk assessment, but he needed to hear what was now known. Eoin was an alcoholic and he had concealed his alcohol consumption with his claim to being a 'man of moderation in most things'.[4]

Would Eoin respond to an open appeal about recovery? We could both acknowledge that in recent years his life and work had been difficult. The stress he felt at work, which depressed him and made him withdraw from his senior role, was paralleled by the stress he felt at home, which made him feel his marriage was in jeopardy. He found that medication was not effective and he wanted a better route to recovery that would include exercise and lifestyle changes. Would he agree to look at all of his lifestyle with an open mind? Could we talk in detail about his use of diet and exercise, recreation and alcohol? On reflection, could we agree that he needed to look at all of these things again?

Eoin was animated. 'You can be a bit more upfront, if you like. What are you really saying? Why are you just skirting around the issues? What has Marion told you about me?'

At this stage it was necessary to be very direct and open with Eoin. I told him that he hadn't been entirely accurate in his descriptions of himself as a man of moderation. I asked him to explain what he meant when he said that he 'liked his pint'. What did that mean? Characteristically, Eoin drew back from our immediate confrontation and he said he would answer truthfully whatever I asked him. Rather than confront each other, we could work together and help with his problems.

The AUDIT or Alcohol Use Disorders Screening Test, developed by the World Health Organization (WHO), is a simple way to screen for excessive drinking and to assist in clinical assessment.[5] According to WHO: '[The test] can help identify excessive drinking as a cause of a presenting illness. It provides a framework for intervention to help risky drinkers reduce or cease harmful alcohol consumption and thereby avoid the harmful consequences of excessive consumption. It helps to identify alcohol dependence and some specific consequences of harmful levels of drinking.'

The questionnaire has three domains identifying: hazardous drinking, harmful drinking and alcohol dependent drinking. Hazardous drinking is indicated by the increasing frequency and increased volume of consumption. Harmful drinking is indicated by the presence of guilt after drinking, lapses in consciousness or memory lapses ('blackouts') associated with alcohol, as well as alcohol-related injuries and expressions of concern from others about the drinking. Dependent drinking is indicated by impaired control over drinking, increased prominence of drink-seeking behaviours and morning drinking for relief from withdrawals. Eoin agreed to go through the audit questions, and this time his answers were much more revealing.

Eoin was drinking at least twice per week and typically he would have five or six drinks each time. One pint is actually two drinks. On a twice-weekly basis, Eoin would have six drinks or more and he had regular episodes where he found it hard to stop drinking. On these occasions he had not been able to do what he was supposed to do, because of the alcohol consumption. Eoin denied that he had an alcohol problem and he insisted that he had never taken an early morning drink. He did feel guilty and remorseful about his alcohol use and his lying about it. He rationalised these 'white lies' by saying he had some episodes of memory lapse in which he had been unable to recall what had happened the night before – but on closer questioning, it was apparent this had always been because of his drinking. He acknowledged that his wife had asked him repeatedly to stop drinking, but he had always ignored her requests. As Eoin put it: 'I am not harming anyone.'

Eoin's denial is a very common phenomenon. By limiting his definition of dependency to a narrow view of the issues (such as whether or not he needed a 'cure' in the mornings), he was able to ignore all the psychological, behavioural and cognitive features of his dependency, and these were obvious to everyone else. His insistence that he had never harmed anyone was also laden with self-deception and denial.

'No one has ever been harmed by my drinking. I have never risked driving while drunk and I am not physically violent.'

It was clear that it would take some time for Eoin to identify his marital conflict in terms of harm, and he found it hard to see that the injury to his relationship with his wife and his children was directly related to his alcohol abuse. But Eoin did agree to working together to form a plan.

In time, Eoin acknowledged that he had lost control over his alcohol consumption. With his score of 21 on the AUDIT, he was in the dependent range. He admitted that at our first meeting he had been less than forthcoming and he even acknowledged that when he was abstinent, his jealous thoughts disappeared. From now on we had a clear set of goals and targets and the challenge was to help Eoin to engage with these.

Marion was also right. Eoin would have to do the recovering for himself – but, the way she saw it, the prize was very great. Eoin could recover, but only if he stopped drinking. There is a great deal spoken about controlled or moderated drinking but the longitudinal data confirms that abstinence is the only route for recovery from alcohol dependence syndrome. The evidence of the natural history of alcoholism is unequivocal about this, and the experience of Alcoholics Anonymous concurs with this view.

Therapy with a counsellor in the multidisciplinary team would be helpful for Eoin. Attending and becoming a supportive member of Alcoholics Anonymous would probably be the most significant contribution to sobriety that he could make. Sometimes medication to support sobriety can be helpful, but ultimately it is continued sobriety that brings continuing peace. Sustaining that peace requires sustained sobriety. Recovery can be circular.

Eoin is sober now after many months of struggle. He made a choice to recover once the consequences of his drinking became apparent to him and once he was willing to accept help and acknowledge that he had no control over his alcohol use. Eoin's sobriety is a continuing struggle and his craving for alcohol at peak times of stress has been very strong.

Eoin is enjoying his fitness and is engaging again with activities that he had lost sight of for more than three years. Now that he is sober, he no longer suspects his wife of an affair. He realises that he was using their relationship in a distorted way to avoid recognition of his own self-loathing and his own guilt. He has accepted that alcohol has a chemical effect on his brain that makes his jealousy emerge. His recovery is a daily journey and he has recognised that he cannot make it on his own. As Eoin puts it: 'Now I decide each day to take help.'

How is Eoin's change of heart to be explained? None of his recovery has been easy, and his sober journey came after years of disabling alcohol abuse. Things could have been very different, and were he to return to alcohol misuse they would almost certainly deteriorate immediately. His story illustrates some of the complexity of mental health. Sometimes a depression is more than it may seem at first meeting. The key to mental health recovery is personal commitment and sustained engagement with all the means of support. Sustained involvement begins with an assessment that is neither judgemental nor stigmatic, but one that offers persistent hope of recovery as the only authentic goal.

Trust

Oh we've got to trust
one another again
in some essentials.

Not the narrow little
bargaining trust
that says: I'm for you
if you'll be for me. –

But a bigger trust,
a trust of the sun
that does not bother
about moth and rust,
and we see it shining
in one another.

Oh don't you trust me,
don't burden me
with your life and affairs; don't
  thrust me
into your cares.

But I think you may trust
the sun in me
that glows with just
as much glow as you see
in me, and no more.

But if it warms
your heart's quick core
why then trust it, it forms
one faithfulness more.

And be, oh be
a sun to me,
not a weary, insistent
personality

but a sun that shines
and goes dark, but shines
again and entwines
with the sunshine in me

till we both of us
are more glorious
and more sunny.

~

D.H. LAWRENCE

Balance

Each person seeking help has a story, and each story has an objective significance as well as a subjective meaning. There may be collateral contributions from relatives, or professional assessments from nursing, psychology or other team members, but the summation of all this narrative is what clinicians call 'the history'. The view famously expressed by Henry Ford that 'all history is bunk' is as far from a shared interpretation of mental health distress as it is possible to get. The history is the beginning of all objective clinical understanding.

Each of us has a past and a present, a childhood and an adulthood, relationships with one another, and a relationship with ourselves. Our mental health first develops in the midst of these interactions and later adapts as we negotiate life, at the centre of what Aaron Beck called the triad of relationships: with the self, with our world and with our future. By discovering this history, the true nature of mental health distress emerges, with all its complex features: social, psychological and biological. Recognition of an objective reality can be a struggle in mental health disorder, but recovery begins with the sharing of a personal history leading to a care plan and an authentic pathway to wellbeing.

In the early years of my training I remember struggling to learn the skills of history-taking. It seemed to take an age to gather a story. I naively expected the salient features would emerge without the necessity to reorganise them into a useful meaningful formulation. It took time to learn that people do not reveal their stories in a linear way, and I mistakenly saw the history exclusively in terms of the search for a cause of the distress.

Mental health problems are difficult to communicate and it can be painful for patients to articulate their real issues. The value we place on the narrative often reflects our prejudices regarding the basis of mental health disorders, where social and psychological understanding rivals the appreciation of biological process.

Society's recognition of human factors in mental health distress is greatest for what we understand as anxiety, depression and addictive disorders, and here we expect the story to illustrate a causal link and thus bring us a comforting clarity. When it comes to psychotic presentations the value of the human narrative is often dismissed, since we instinctively assume no sense will come from that dialogue.

In truth, the human story in psychosis is just as relevant as it is in other mental health presentations. People in psychosis need communication and enlightened recognition of their problems, and it is a mistake to think of the conversation's value only in terms of our search for the cause of mental health distress.

Dialogue is essentially humane, and continued engagement and communication over time is essential for recovery and maintenance of wellbeing. Sometimes the last thing that is said turns out to be the most significant of all.

Kathleen

Patients with a manic psychosis may need admission to hospital for intensive treatment in an area dedicated to their care. The simple measure of reducing the amount of visual and auditory stimulation in the environment can have a beneficial calming effect, minimising some of the chaos of psychotic thinking and limiting disorganised behaviour. Higher levels of nursing and professional care may be necessary for the safe use of specific therapies including antipsychotic medication and psychotherapy. The special care unit at St Patrick's University Hospital is an example of such an intensive care area where nurses and staff specialise in the recovery of patients with psychosis.

One day I was sitting in the special care unit listening to a woman whose thoughts and behaviour were very disorganised by a manic psychosis. Her story appeared to be going nowhere, and so after a while we agreed to end our conversation. Despite her distraction, she was thankful for our meeting. As she went to the door, she turned back and said: 'By the way, doctor, did I ever tell you that my mother was a fish?'

It took a moment to know how to react, but then it became clear. Our meeting had not ended; in fact, our conversation had just begun.

Later, Kathleen told me her story. 'My name is Kathleen and I have had two dramatic mental breakdowns. On the most recent occasion, I left home with my husband's credit card and I booked myself in to one of Dublin's most exclusive hotels.

'I was quite certain at the time that I had a mission to house the poor of Dublin. And it seemed that a city centre hotel was as good a place as any to base my campaign. Once I was in the hotel, I gathered as many people as I could in the foyer. I arranged to bring them to my suite and we ordered champagne and room service. Looking back, one thing is obvious to me: I certainly know how to throw a good party!'

Kathleen described her manic episode in more detail.[1]

'I had been developing these grandiose plans over a period of about a fortnight. During that time, I had no apparent need for sleep. By the time I booked myself into the hotel, I was in very poor shape. I had telephoned a number of charities asking them to send homeless people to my hotel suite, where I could care for them.

'I alerted many people to my plans, but no one responded. I suppose they considered it to be rather a bizarre initiative. That was why I resorted to going to the hotel foyer to ask complete strangers up to my room. I thought I had some sort of gift and that I could rehouse the needy and the dispossessed.

'Then, when I discovered that many of the "guests" in my room were neither impoverished nor homeless, I became acutely agitated and angry with them. My charity initiative was brought to an end when the hotel management realised what was really going on.'

Prior to her admission Kathleen had been having a very difficult year with numerous episodes of depression and frequent hypomanic episodes. She met criteria for a particularly challenging form of the disorder known as rapid cycling bipolar mood disorder. Convention regards this disorder as being present when four or more mood episodes occur within a twelve-month period. Further treatment with antidepressant medication may actually worsen this variant of the disorder. That is one of the reasons why proper assessment is necessary when treating recurrent or resistant mood disorders. Women with bipolar mood disorder are more likely to suffer in this way and physical factors such as poor thyroid function and menopausal or menstrual cycle irregularities seem to be contributory.[2]

Kathleen had normal thyroid function but she was going through the menopause. Most of her previous mood episodes had been depressive in nature but her recent depressions had been agitated and restless. Some time later, Kathleen and I met to discuss her progress. She described her experience fluently in her own terms.

'When I was unwell I had restless energy and not sadness. I woke up in the morning and I was agitated and so I became full of distress and unease. What I had was something that might be better described as "motorised misery" and that is not what I call depression. My agitation actually got worse on some of the medications. I needed the doctors to understand that my illness does its own thing.'

The core of treatment for bipolar mood disorder is pharmacological; that is to say, it requires medication to stabilise mood, reduce mania and minimise depression. Essentially, the frequency of mood shifts needs to be reduced and the most effective way of doing this is through mood-stabilising treatments and not antidepressants.

Lithium is a mood stabiliser and 50 per cent of bipolar patients will benefit from it. Unfortunately, lithium is not usually effective in rapid cycling mood disorder. There are other mood stabilisers, and each of these medications has its own set of side effects and hazards requiring close medical monitoring in general practice or in a mental health clinic.

Lithium is associated with risks to thyroid and kidney function and these hazards need to be limited by maintaining the blood level of the drug within very narrow limits. There may also be significant risks to the foetus in pregnant bipolar women being treated with these drugs so these real dangers also need to be managed with care.

Kathleen has made a very good recovery. Her psychosis has disappeared completely, as gradually her antidepressant treatment was withdrawn and replaced with mood-stabilising alternatives.

Her agitation was reduced with the addition of an antipsychotic. Unfortunately, she gained considerable weight on this medicine and she became distressed by this and so this too was gradually withdrawn.

For Kathleen, the introduction of a mood stabilising medicine over time was associated with definite and sustained reduction in the turbulence of her mood. With gradual withdrawal of the antipsychotic, she agreed a new lifestyle programme. With diet and exercise, Kathleen regained her healthy weight and made steady progress over the weeks and months following her stay in hospital.

I had an interesting conversation with Kathleen in my room at a later date. She explained: 'I really wish the doctors had heard me earlier and recognised more quickly that I was not depressed. Eventually my agitation was understood and now I am on a new plan. It is not easy to communicate these things, but when I did get things across, that message got me on the right road.'

'And what about the time you said your mother was a fish?' I asked.

Kathleen responded hesitantly: 'You know, I have no recollection of ever saying that to you. So who knows what I meant at the time? I must have been very unwell.'

Then she smiled and said: 'On reflection, maybe it did mean something to me at the time... After all, my mother was a Pisces!'

We were both amused at this insight – and we laughed for some time.

Kathleen remains well.

Up-Hill

Does the road wind up-hill all the way?
   Yes, to the very end.
Will the day's journey take the whole long day?
   From morn to night, my friend.

But is there for the night a resting-place?
   A roof for when the slow dark hours begin.
May not the darkness hide it from my face?
   You cannot miss that inn.

Shall I meet other wayfarers at night?
   Those who have gone before.
Then must I knock, or call when just in sight?
   They will not keep you standing at that door.

Shall I find comfort, travel-sore and weak?
   Of labor you shall find the sum.
Will there be beds for me and all who seek?
   Yea, beds for all who come.

CHRISTINA ROSSETTI

Andrew

A ndrew is tall and lean with a fit physique and a full head of dark hair. He is married with two grown-up daughters. One afternoon he stood in my room and told me that he had invented a very special piece of computer software that was going to revolutionise the movement of goods and packages around the world. He was very emphatic about the subject; in his view, his invention would make millions for his family and for Ireland.

'After the fall of the Celtic Tiger, my invention could restart the nation's economy. And I have the vision and the connections to see it through. I could get the right kind of people to support my plans.'

At first, Andrew refused to sit down as he was very reluctant to rest. As far as he was concerned he was in a hurry and he had things to do. He spoke quickly but in a soft voice, almost whispering at times, and then dramatically laughing out loud when least expected. As he paced my room, he suddenly turned and held out his hand to feel the end of my necktie. He admired its colours and then started to ask me some questions about my life.

'Tell me,' he said, 'did you always want to be a psychiatrist?'

'No,' I replied, 'for many years I was unsure about my career.'

'Aha!' he replied. 'You were in two minds! That is the perfect state of mind for a psychiatrist!' He laughed out heartily.

Without any prompting, Andrew returned to his earlier theme and explained how he would get the major funding needed to develop his invention and regenerate our economy.

Then he said, 'I cannot talk about this now. You and I need to go for a walk – a long walk. What I need to know right now is this:

are you going to help me out? Or are you just going to sit there and waste my time?'

It seemed reasonable to try to put Andrew at his ease and to allow him some space to share his story. Perhaps then he would allow me to assess his mental state and make a diagnosis. Instead, Andrew became more irritable. He dismissed even the mildest reassurances and gentlest of questions.

'I really insist that you come for a walk. We can talk – alright? But we can only do that if we go outside. Come on outside. Let's get some of the evening air. Let's look at this city that I'm going to regenerate!'

It was impossible to decline Andrew's invitation. He was dismissive until I agreed to leave the room with him. Luckily there was no one else waiting outside. Rather than have a row, it seemed best to agree to go with him for a walk up James's Street. As we made our way past the Guinness Brewery towards Thomas Street and Christchurch, Andrew's pace increased and it was harder to keep up with him.

Andrew's safety and his privacy were my major concerns, as it seemed inevitable that others would notice us. His bodily behaviour was very energetic, and the rate of his speech was greatly increased, but Andrew was utterly unconcerned as he continued to pace at speed disregarding any possible intrusion from anyone who might be listening to him.

His speech was rapid and rambling with multiple side remarks and digressions. His narrative was impossible to direct or to follow, but we continued together on our brisk walk past John's Lane Church towards Cornmarket. By the time we got to the junction with Francis Street, I was out of breath. At my request, Andrew agreed to stop for a while at a little coffee shop on the corner. As we went in to the coffee shop, Andrew immediately ordered two large coffees and a plate of buns and insisted that we were to have as much as we wanted to eat.

Andrew talked on and on. Throughout this time he was smiling and charming, but also intrusive in all of his interactions with the staff and other people in the coffee shop. He shifted back and forth with casual irritability.

'I have always had extraordinary vision and an ability to understand great concepts. What we need today is energy and I have that in spades. That is why I love my work. It is energy that has made me so successful. Energy.'

We sat over our coffee and buns and Andrew continued to talk at galloping speed until he stopped quite suddenly and whispered: 'Well, are you going to help me, or are you not?'

By now I had formed the opinion that Andrew was suffering from a manic episode.[1]

Andrew repeatedly asked me about my family background and then he offered information about his own. 'Both of my parents are dead. Yes. They divorced when I was ten. I knew little of my father growing up. My mother and grandparents raised me. I had one older brother. He went into the defence forces. We weren't really in contact, although I learned a few years ago that he took his own life. My mother called me. He was found dead, hanging at the barracks. She was very sad. There was no explanation. Well, you know how these things go. I'm sure it was all for the best, really. What were you like growing up? I was very popular and I was very good at sports. I wasn't what you'd call academic.'

I asked Andrew what he thought might be done for him. At first he didn't answer. Then he responded angrily.

'Don't you *understand*? I am not looking for any counselling here. I am offering to cut you in at the conceptual phase of a major technological development that will transform our economy and create thousands of jobs for the city of Dublin. Do you get that? In the past few weeks I have met the Dalai Lama and President Bill Clinton and they are totally behind the whole innovation. What we are going to do is bring to Dublin a new generation concept, with unprecedented environmental functionality that works at political, spiritual and psychological levels. It's going to revolutionise the way we think and live and work in the city.'

Andrew acknowledged that recently he had not been sleeping well but he insisted that he wasn't tired and that he felt 'great'. He said his thoughts were especially clear and his capacity to get things done had never been greater. It was obvious that his motor activity was heightened and his judgement was now distorted with grandiose plans. It wasn't possible to know whether Andrew had ever been depressed or suicidal in the past. Now, as far as could be seen in the coffee shop, Andrew was a man experiencing a severe manic episode.

I tried to tell him that I would help him. In my view he needed an entirely different kind of help to the one he was requesting from me. Suddenly Andrew became very angry with me and he insisted that I was being unhelpful. Then he rounded on me.

'You really are screwing things up! I *knew* it was a mistake to tell you about the Dalai Lama and Bill Clinton. That's why you don't believe me, isn't it? You are wrong, you know. Both of them have been in Dublin recently and I have seen them, but you just think I am talking some kind of paranoid nonsense. That's the problem with psychiatrists. They just don't know what to believe. I shouldn't have trusted you, but it is my mistake. I was trying to do you a favour. Believe me, it's not an error I will make again.'

Andrew rose to his full height and leaned over the table, talking in a determined voice with his face up close to mine.

'I hoped you would help me, but now I see this is what you are really like. This has been an utter waste of my time as far as I am concerned. Thank you very much. Goodbye.'

After that, Andrew strode out of the coffee shop and walked briskly towards the city centre. I was stunned for a few moments. As I paid the bill at the counter, I wondered how I might have handled things differently. I walked outside and turned back up Thomas

Street towards the hospital. I decided to make an urgent call to the office of Andrew's GP.

Andrew's GP was very concerned. He had treated Andrew twice before for depressive episodes, but as far as we knew this was the first time Andrew had experienced a manic one. The GP said that Andrew had been a cause for concern for the past three weeks, after being very down in mood for some months. Andrew's wife had made some very distressed calls to the GP practice and she had hoped that he would agree to take some treatment. Unfortunately, in the coffee shop we did not get anywhere near agreeing a treatment plan, let alone come to an agreed understanding of the nature of Andrew's problems. Both myself and the GP recognised that Andrew needed help, but we had hoped he would agree to take help voluntarily.

Things took their course rapidly and dramatically after our meeting in the coffee shop. Andrew's wife was horrified when she returned home to find her husband in the bath attempting to end his life. She immediately called an ambulance and Andrew agreed to come into hospital. Andrew was a very unwell man and he needed urgent care. His safety was our immediate priority and the treatment of his mood disorder was now an urgent necessity in hospital.

This was Andrew's first time in hospital and much depended on the quality of this experience. His physical wounds would heal quickly enough, but his mental pain would require a greater understanding and more time. When he came to us the day of his suicide attempt, he was distressed but his manic features had already begun to elide. His awareness of his plight was increasing but he was already expressing regret for what he had done, even if he did not yet understand the connection between his mood swings and his behaviour.

During his stay in hospital, Andrew assured us of his safety. For the first hours and days of his care he was treated with a high level of observation and extra vigilance. Gradually we worked out an individual care plan that included progress towards recovery in stages, initially with a period emphasising stabilisation of his mood. This included nursing and medical support. Later, we introduced occupational therapy and therapeutic education about his diagnosis. Over the following two weeks, we established his treatment with a mood-stabilising medication and transferred him to outpatient care. Thankfully, Andrew has since made a good recovery.

Andrew's wife has been very supportive and she has seen him work hard to maintain a programme that gets him well and keeps him well. Andrew himself is keen on adjunctive treatments also. We have been open and supportive of his search for a range of recovery options built around (rather than as an alternative to) his treatment plan. Andrew attends a counsellor who is a psychologist in his community and Andrew follows up with our mood disorder group at our Dean Clinic. Andrew likes to take omega-3 fatty acids along with his lithium, which is being monitored on a monthly basis. His psychotherapy emphasises the importance of interpersonal and family relationships and he has found it helpful to see his mood disorder in the context of his social life.

Andrew is keen on the idea of becoming an advocate for mental health recovery, an 'expert by experience'. For now, though, he wants to move on, to get well and to stay well. We spoke recently and he had this to say: 'When I was very unwell, my life was fantastic and unreal. In my manic time I had great dreams and schemes, but I now understand that they were part of a long nightmare. I am hoping my recovered life will be less extraordinary. In fact, I would be quite happy with that.'

The Lake Isle of Innisfree

I will arise and go now, and go to Innisfree,
And a small cabin build there, of clay and wattles made:
Nine bean-rows will I have there, a hive for the honey-bee,
And live alone in the bee-loud glade.

And I shall have some peace there, for peace comes dropping slow,
Dropping from the veils of the morning to where the cricket sings;
There midnight's all a glimmer, and noon a purple glow,
And evening full of the linnet's wings.

I will arise and go now, for always night and day
I hear lake water lapping with low sounds by the shore;
While I stand on the roadway, or on the pavements grey,
I hear it in the deep heart's core.

∼

W.B. YEATS

Hope

When someone dies by suicide, the bereaved experience unimaginable pain. The suffering of the living is beyond words, and beyond comparison. However well we may have known the person, it is never possible to predict when death is going to happen, and so the suicide comes as a terrible shock. For those bereaved as a result of an accident or a catastrophic injury, death also comes as a shock, but the tangible causes of death are evident to everyone and those in mourning have some form of explanation. After suicide we are left with so many unanswered questions. The sense of loss is fused with feelings of anger, regret and guilt, and these shared anxieties are amplified in the tormented grief of the intimately bereaved as they seek vainly for answers with which to carry on.

Data from the World Health Organization tells us that approximately one million people worldwide die by suicide every year. This translates as one death by suicide every 40 seconds. None of us knows why any particular person has taken their own life and no one can say who will take this final step. Suicide cannot be predicted with certainty or prevented with absolute confidence. So it remains an enigma to us, even if it is frequently recognised as the catastrophic consequence of psychological pain, intoxication and despair. We do know that in most suicides mental health has been lost leading up to the final act of hopelessness. And yet, experience teaches us that mental wellbeing might have been restored with the right help.

Death by suicide is more than a daily occurrence in Ireland. Since 1990 there has been a four-fold increase in the number of these deaths and suicide has become the commonest cause of death of our young people. Each catastrophic loss is more painfully tragic because it seems so often that it could have been prevented.

The most compelling data on suicide in Ireland comes from the work of Professor Kevin Malone of the Department of Psychiatry at University College Dublin. Supported by funding from a number of charitable organisations such as the 3Ts (Turning The Tide Against Suicide), Professor Malone and his colleagues have produced a comprehensive review called *Suicide in Ireland 2003–2008*. Their data reveal that when all age groups are combined, the suicide rate per year in Ireland for the past two decades has been approximately 8.2/100,000, ranking Ireland at number 18 out of 25 European Union states. However, youth suicide rates (suicide in those under 25 years of age) have steadily increased in Ireland since the late 1980s, so that the most recent complete WHO data (2009) indicates that Ireland has the fourth highest youth suicide rate in the expanded European Union. The annual level is 14.4/100,000, which lies behind the youth suicide rates of Lithuania, Estonia and Finland. By combining the total number of definite and probable suicides (including those deaths given an open verdict at the Coroner's Court in Ireland) the actual total was 722 in 2009 and this is much higher than the official figure of 510 for that same year. As the Malone report puts it: 'On average, every 18 days a child under 18 dies by suicide in Ireland.'

At least three factors contribute to the problem of suicide: mental health disorder, alcohol abuse and, lastly, what Professor Malone calls an 'Ireland factor' that is as yet undefined. It is a matter of speculation as to what is included under this last cultural heading, but the important thing is to recognise that suicide is a cultural phenomenon influenced by collective societal factors as well as individual personal pain. Youth unemployment and the loss of social cohesion that is common to our modern environment are acknowledged cultural factors particularly associated with youth suicide.

Suicidal ideas are probably universal at times of great distress. Although they are not in themselves indicative of mental disorder, they are much more frequent within it. They may not represent a functional adaptation to any circumstance, but they are usually an indication of the scale of the distress and of the mental pain of the patient. Suicide has to be acknowledged, but this recognition of suicide neither normalises it nor idealises it. Acknowledgment is necessary so that we can begin to understand.

For some people the idea of suicide as a possible solution to their suffering can be comforting in times of extreme distress. Severe depression is an experience in which deep personal pain is sometimes unbearable. While a person may not ever intend to die by suicide, some of those suffering from overwhelming levels of depression may feel relieved by the thought that they could, after all, take control. Suicide becomes a means of escape; a way of ending their pain completely.

This leaves us with a dilemma. How should we respond when our community is struck by suicide? There is no clear answer. While we must try to avoid doing anything which adds to suffering, we all need to be able to talk about suicide without a fear that we will be punished or dismissed or silenced. If we can talk about the symptoms we may be able to appreciate the small clues, the subtle (and not so subtle) hints that may escape us when we are doing our daily battle with life.

A patient of mine, Eddie, regularly tells me about his suicidal ideas and then just as quickly insists that he would never do it to himself. One day in my room, Eddie described his suicidal feelings in this way.

'It is like a car crash going on inside me. I have a physical sense of being torn apart from the inside; like a physical wrenching within

me. My senses move into total darkness, and my loss of hope is
absolute as well as a loss of the ability to connect with anything or
anybody. I experience a feeling that nobody can or will ever want to
connect with me again.'

Eddie then went on to say: 'Still, at least I can tell you about
my suicide thoughts because I know you don't overreact. If I told
others they would probably have me admitted to a secure ward and
I would have to stay quiet about my ideas until they let me out
again.'

There is something counterintuitive about what Eddie is
saying. It seems paradoxical that he only feels able to talk about
his suicidal symptoms when he is confident that an emergency
response is unlikely. In an ideal reciprocal therapeutic relationship,
a patient would be respected as a whole person, rather than a set
of symptoms or hazards potentially warranting an emergency
reaction. Mental health risk assessment is best when it is based upon
an understanding of the patient's whole mental state and when
patients are able to tell their symptoms without fear of negative
consequences.

Of course I have not given Eddie a guarantee about the response
to his suicidal symptoms; but the fact is that Eddie has repeatedly
given me his guarantee of safety and that is far more valuable. For
as long as possible, we will both have to rely on that. In treating
Eddie's depression, we have been able to talk frequently about his
suicidal ideas and no suicidal action has taken place. Sitting in my
room, Eddie described his suicidal suffering.

'One of the worst parts of having a mental illness is the periods
that you go through when you have lost control of your life and
have, in effect, ceded it to the illness. You feel that you have no
options and that you cannot make choices. It may sound bizarre
but there is a relief in simply having the concept that, if you wanted
to, you could end your own life – that you do have options and
that you can make choices. For the time being, you choose life –

however miserable and unbearable it might feel at times. Reaching this conclusion means having one less argument with myself and one less battle to fight for the day.

'I know that the fact of having suicidal thoughts is perceived as "wrong" and "bad", and so whenever I experience these ideas I get even more distressed. Perhaps because of this I turn further inwards, and I can become completely unable to talk to anyone. In my distress, what little I have left of myself is destroyed and I move closer to the abyss. It is no good for me to live in fear of my suicidal thoughts – or of other people's judgement about them.'

Talking about suicide does not make it happen, but suppressing the conversation may do. What is more, any therapeutic dialogue needs to be dynamic since its context may change over time. We need to be able to have the discussion so that we can recognise these changing circumstances. When suicide is spoken of as an item on a possible future agenda, its resonance may be weaker and its immediate hazard may be lower. When it becomes proximal and spoken of with morbid features such as the planning of the specific means of death and the finalisation of life's affairs (the arrangement of the so-called 'last acts'), it may be more indicative of jeopardy. In order to have any chance of recognising this subtle morbid shift when it occurs, it is essential that assessments happen regularly. It is a tragedy that anyone should ever end his or her own life without having the opportunity for this conversation.

Intoxication seems to be a universal enabler of suicide and occasionally a direct cause. Alcohol generates depressive ideas and destructive behaviours, but it also dulls the pain of melancholy and stops self-reasoning in its tracks. Destructive actions are easier to make when the handbrake of inhibition is released. Equally, the evidence is that completed suicide is most frequently a consequence of extreme mental distress and despair, whether this is with or without intoxication. The most likely correlate of this despair is clinical depression.

Treatment for depression can be effective even for those who experience a sense of profound hopelessness. Despite life's absurdity, most people with depressive disorder do recover. This perennial buoyancy speaks in part to the remarkable resilience of the human spirit; and therein lays a hidden truth.

Mrs Jones and her grandson Paul

One day while sitting in my room I received an unexpected phone call. The switchboard said: 'You have a call from Mr Jones.' I asked them to hold the call for a few moments before I responded, so that I could gather my thoughts and consider what I should say.

It had been four years since I had last seen Mr Jones in the aftermath of his wife's tragic death. Mrs Jones hanged herself one Saturday evening in the spring of the year 2000 while her husband was at Mass and only one week after I had seen her for the very first time.

The mixture of thoughts going through my mind was briefly overpowering. I could remember the shock of hearing about her death and the sadness of her grief-stricken family after the terrible news, as they described their pain at the loss of a loving wife, a beloved mother and a gentle grandmother.

Mrs Jones had been the matriarchal head of a caring family. Any words at the time of her death seemed to be of little use. There was no doubt that she had been very unwell. Her clinical depression had been obvious at our only meeting. In truth, the full degree of her despair had not been apparent, even though there was sufficient concern to recommend that she come into hospital for treatment.

I remembered my meeting with Mrs Jones very clearly. She had come to my room urgently one afternoon, accompanied by her husband and their three adult daughters. I remember asking to speak with Mrs Jones on my own, but all of the family responded by insisting that I should not do so. Mrs Jones said that she wanted her husband and her daughters to remain with her throughout our meeting. She said that she would prefer it that way, and so she asked earnestly that we proceed as she wished, with her family still present.

On assessment, it was clear she was in the depths of a severe depressive episode with clinical melancholic features that required urgent treatment. Access to her old notes revealed her clinical record. Some years earlier, she had a similar depressive episode also with biological features. On that occasion, according to our records, she had responded very well to treatment. This time, just as before, she complained of low mood, with broken sleep and early morning wakening. She spoke about her variation of mood throughout the day, with mornings that were very bleak and evenings that were a little brighter. As in the earlier episode, her mental concentration had decreased substantially so that she found thinking very difficult and she was moving much more slowly than before. She had lost her appetite and more than 7 kg in weight. Despite all these clinical features, Mrs Jones denied any risk to herself and she rejected any suggestion that admission to hospital was warranted for inpatient treatment or for her safety.

With all of these memories flooding my mind, I asked for the call to be put through to my room.

'Hello, Mr Jones. How can I help you?'

…

'Yes, of course I remember you. How could I forget?'

…

'Yes, this is a good time for me to talk. Is it a good time for you?'

…

'Of course, I would be happy to meet with you and with your daughters at any time. Let's arrange a meeting soon.'

We met early the very next week. When the Jones family arrived in my room they were obviously distressed but, to my great relief, there was no trace of any anger in their approach. They explained that they had come seeking help and they wanted to tell something about their late mother; something they felt must come out sooner or later. They had a secret they needed to share. For everyone's sake, it needed to be told.

It was this. They had known their mother was having suicidal thoughts but they had agreed to be bound to secrecy since she made this a condition when she agreed to come to see a psychiatrist. The family had been desperate to get their mother to have treatment, and she had repeatedly refused their earlier requests. In her last brief intense depressive episode, she had insisted that no one should know of her problems. And so the family had to agree to keep her morbid ideas a secret from her GP. These were her terms. These were her conditions before agreeing to come to see any psychiatrist. At that time, it seemed to the family that this was the only way they could proceed.

I asked why the family had insisted on staying with Mrs Jones during our only meeting. Mr Jones spoke: 'She insisted that we all come together. I think she wanted to be sure that nobody would break the agreement and say anything that she didn't want the doctors to hear.'

Was Mrs Jones by nature a suspicious or controlling woman?

'Goodness, no,' Mr Jones said. 'She was none of those things. She was a lovely woman. So gentle in nature – a very gentle presence in our home. But she was quite stubborn about this issue. It was out of character, really. We never saw that until she became unwell.'

Had she been otherwise well for much of her life?

Mr Jones spoke. 'She was – but things became very complicated when she got low that first time. She had a bad experience of depression that time. It really was dreadful for her.

'She got treatment and she got well. She really did recover well. But the fear was always there. She had this desperate fear of ever becoming ill again. She didn't speak much about it – never to the girls. But she'd say things to me the odd time and I could tell how much it weighed on her mind.

'She would make me promise that I would never have her admitted or treated against her will. Usually I was able to reassure her, to talk her round. The topic would pass, but then…it might be a year or so later, and it would come up again. The second time she got ill there was nothing I could say to reassure her. Nothing.

'In the end, I decided to tell the girls. I was desperate. I had to tell them. By now, they were grown women, so I thought it was the right thing to do.

'But my wife couldn't forgive me for breaking that secret. She saw her illness as a weakness, and she was so upset that I told the girls about it. Of course, the girls saw that we were dealing with a serious situation. Once they knew, things moved on quickly after that. That's how we came here the first time.'

Mrs Jones had refused to go to her GP, but she had agreed to see a psychiatrist because a predecessor of mine had been her psychiatrist when she had her first serious depression and, in truth, she had made a great recovery on that occasion. Mr Jones explained that his wife had been very quick to respond to treatment on the previous episode, and that she also got on very well with her psychiatrist. The original psychiatrist had since retired and so the family were given my name instead.

Mr Jones spoke at length about all that had happened in the intervening years. 'We just feel her absence so painfully. It is constant. Even sitting here now, it's obvious that there's one less person in the room. It's very hard to come to terms with it. She ended her life before anyone could really help her.

'We need to explain to you, doctor, why we've come back now. We haven't really come to see you about my late wife, as such. Our real worry is my grandson Paul.'

Mr Jones turned to one of his daughters and he invited her to speak. 'Why don't you tell the doctor why we are here?'

And so Paul's mother spoke, as we all listened in earnest.

'I'm Eileen – and Paul is my son. He is a lovely boy. You would expect me to say that about him, wouldn't you? After all, I am his mother. But it is true: he is really a fine young man. Paul was 16 when his Granny died. And they had been really close all through the years. Now he's in college. His real interest is in computers. Unfortunately, last year his girlfriend broke up with him and since then he has been going downhill. We thought it was a normal thing that he just had to go through. Everyone has their heart broken at some stage in their life, don't they? But Paul has continued to go steadily down ever since then.

'I suppose it's been tough for him coming on top of the loss of his grandmother. I don't think he's ever come to terms with that. He hasn't had it easy. Now it's more than just the break-up. He has lost all interest in life and he seems to have lost all of his sense of fun. He has no energy. It's a struggle for him to get up and out of bed at all.

'You see, his Granny was very important to him. When his father and I divorced, he was only a child. He and his Granny were very close. They did so much together. She practically raised him, when I think back on it. She loved to talk about GAA with him and they'd go to Croke Park together during the summer. She was a great woman for playing golf as well. They were never short of things to talk about.

'I've told Paul that his Granny died by suicide. He was at an age where he knew what was going on. But I think he has never understood why his Granny left him in the way that she did. What can we say to him now? He still knows nothing about her mental health problems.

'We feel guilty enough about our mother's death, but we all worry that Paul will become unwell in the same way. Now we are very afraid it will end with the same result and so we are looking for answers and we need some help. What should we do for Paul now?'

Is there a right response to the bereaved? Is it best to avoid the risk of burdening the anguished with advice, and better instead to reply that in death there are no simple answers? Some might say that any response could run the risk of sounding glib and making a bad situation even worse, by giving answers that were mere opinions and directing the Jones family down one or other ill-defined or unjustified route. What good would that do? On the other hand, surely it was essential to be kind to them and to respond to them with complete honesty.

I asked them to forgive me if I spoke about these things in a seemingly clinical way. Knowing that anything I said might be upsetting for them, I told them that I would answer any question they had for me and give them any answers I could, and so we went ahead.

'I want to tell you', I said, 'that I am deeply sorry for your loss. It seems to me that despite what happened to Mrs Jones you must try to remember her now and always the way that she was when she was well and living life to the full, achieving all the things you loved her for, being a wife, a mother and grandmother. Nothing that she accomplished in her life can be diminished by her suicide. Your love for her and your affectionate memory of her achievements must remain intact, regardless of the manner of her death.

'Eileen, your son Paul has had his heart broken at least three times in a very short life. From what you have told me, the loss of his grandmother may have been the biggest heartbreak. He may not know that his Granny became very unwell. She had a severe recurrent depressive disorder and her symptoms were not explicable in purely social or psychological or biological terms. Her depression was not her fault, but neither was it yours or Paul's.

'Clinical depression is a brain disorder. Paul needs to know that his Granny was overwhelmed by this disorder in the same way that someone might be struck with a cancer or another terminal physical illness, and so she was swept away.

'Speaking about the chemical nature of her depressive disorder is not to disregard the many complex factors that contributed to the development of her clinical depression. The division of causes for depression into social, psychological or biological strands is artificial – and this division helps only those advocates with opposing political or ideological intentions. Sadly, mental health is still full of such fictional disagreement, but a humane understanding of depression is not based on any theory of blame, but on the integration of all the clinical evidence that exists.

'Multiple chemical abnormalities occur in people with severe depression. The function of brain chemical messengers (such as serotonin) is decreased. Key brain structures involved in the regulation of mood (such as the hippocampus) are reduced in size, and the level of the stress hormone cortisol is elevated to such a degree that the size of the adrenal glands is greatly increased. Whether these phenomena are cause or effect is debatable, but the distressing experience for the patient is undoubtedly very real. It is very complex.'

Mr Jones spoke at this point. 'Yes, it is very complex. There are explanations – and then there's understanding. It is very hard for us to come to any understanding about this. My wife wasn't under any particular stress. Our lives were good. Our family was well. We lived for each other… and so I cannot understand it.'

Mr Jones was right too. Many people are unable to locate an environmental stress-related reason for their depression, and for them there is no direct connection between personal suffering and the events in a life. Mrs Jones's life had been good, but she still succumbed to severe depression. Her condition might have been reversed with treatment, and recovery might have been possible, since we know she made a good response to treatment before.

Mr Jones was weeping now and I was very concerned as to how best to continue our meeting. Then Eileen spoke again: 'If all that is the case, doctor, then what is to be done about my Paul?'

Symptoms of a prolonged grief reaction are very similar to

depression and they may co-exist with a depressive episode. Clearly, Paul needed an assessment and expert help. And Paul's family needed to know that he could be well. Eileen felt the added shame arising from her stigmatic belief that Paul's suffering must have been handed down through her genes. Her self-stigma arose from a mistaken sense of inevitability, coming from the belief that genes are all-powerful forces determining rather than merely influencing the outcome of our lives.

It was important to reassure Eileen. Family studies do show an increased familial risk of developing depressive disorder and the earlier the age of onset, the higher the familial risk. But in terms of mode of inheritance there is no compelling evidence of direct transfer. Neither is it possible to be categorical about social, biological or inherited origins for the depressive disorder. The evidence suggests there are significant familial components to both the tendency to experience adverse life events and the tendency to become depressed in response to them. Many factors contribute to the development of depression and each can be seen as contributing at different levels.

Paul's family needed to believe in recovery. We concluded our meeting by agreeing to offer Paul a plan. It would be important to respect Paul's autonomy, but to offer him an assessment based on the awareness of the necessity of early intervention. If there is a familial basis for the risk of depression it seems to be in the inherited predisposition to become depressed in response to life events. Three-quarters of adults with mental health disorders such as depression had their first illness before the age of 24. With early intervention, the potential for kindling a succession of depressive episodes is reduced and the prospect of sustained recovery is increased.

Eileen agreed to ask Paul to visit his GP. Paul did this, and he also agreed to an assessment in our Dean Clinic. Later, he attended our young adult programme for a while as a day patient. He has received counselling for his grief and loss. These were major factors in his suffering and he has benefited from acknowledgement of them, as well as effective intervention for them.

I haven't seen the Jones family together since – but Eileen rang me one day out of the blue. She told me that Paul has been doing well. He is still at college and he is well on the road to recovery. His life can now prosper without the despair of untreated depression or the stigmatic burden of its denial.

Pain Has an Element of Blank

Pain has an element of blank;
It cannot recollect
When it began, or if there were
A day when it was not.

It has no future but itself,
Its infinite realms contain
Its past, enlightened to perceive
New periods of pain.

~

EMILY DICKINSON

Hope is the Thing with Feathers

Hope is the thing with feathers
That perches in the soul,
And sings the tune without the words,
And never stops at all,

And sweetest in the gale is heard;
And sore must be the storm
That could abash the little bird
That kept so many warm.

I've heard it in the chillest land,
And on the strangest sea;
Yet, never, in extremity,
It asked a crumb of me.

~

EMILY DICKINSON

Possibilities

A healthy mind sustains our wellbeing, because it integrates the real markers of mental health: our abilities to live, to work and to love. With mental distress and disorder, the coherence of these human functions is interrupted at least for a time. In reality not even the most resilient of human beings maintains these functions optimally throughout all of a life, and it is true to say that almost anyone can break down at times of great personal stress.

The universal challenge of recovery can be compared to the circus act in which a performer tries to spin numerous plates on the tops of sticks. For a while, the performer keeps a number of plates spinning – but as the demand increases and time passes, the plates begin to fall to the ground. Usually at this point in the circus act a smiling assistant is called upon to help and together they work at making all the plates spin once again. Eventually, even with assistance, the performance comes to its close. In life, as in the circus, mental health involves a willingness to accept this inevitable closure. Resilience in the face of stress requires the capacity to respond even to the most unwelcome challenges. This final adaptation is an essential part of mental health and with maturity it becomes an important pillar of recovery: the ability to accept the ultimate human reality.

The recovery philosophy is obviously appropriate from a human rights perspective but the evidence of its clinical efficacy is also a justification for the recovery approach. Recovery is more than a historical critique of mental health services of the past. It is a philosophy promoting personal wellness, and a testimony to the ability of human beings to build a meaningful and fulfilled life even after a period of mental distress or disorder. Seen in this way, recovery may not be an abrupt event but a gradual and continuing process, and one that thrives in an atmosphere of openness to a variety of methods and a diversity of approaches to mental health care. Recovery of this kind becomes a personal journey sustained by hope, focused on wellness rather than illness, and without predetermined limits, apart from those set by the unique potential of each individual.

Recovery is worthwhile even if mental health problems recur at some later stage, and recovery is facilitated where there is belief in the possibility of becoming well once again. This may seem naïve, since a hopeful sense of expectation is one of the first cognitions to be tested in depression. But all of the evidence points to the fact that true recovery occurs far more frequently than was once believed, and recovery is more likely where this potential is credited by all involved. Hope is therapeutic. In the past, the institutional view of mental problems was filled with pessimism, but a modern service promoting a recovery ethos will have greater inclusion and empowerment of each patient. The recovery journey can be one of discovery, enhancing new skills for living and amplifying new strategies to rebuild a more secure self.

So what is the secret to a successful recovery? To paraphrase Professor George Vaillant of Harvard University, it is in our 'adaptation to life'. Many recovered patients become 'experts by experience', possessed of a new and sustaining wisdom born of real mental health challenge. This exceptional expertise can include a deeper understanding of personal stresses and a willingness to make functional changes in lifestyle and attitude. In a recovery-based mental health service the capacity to make these decisions about one's mental health is not just assumed: it is supported. Fully informed and fully respected patients can choose to take effective measures including engagement with various psychotherapies and/

or specific medications. When these interventions are offered and there is evidence to support their effectiveness, recovery progresses and the full evidence of therapeutic risk and effectiveness is made available to the patient. Personal choice and informed capacity determine the way forward. The best recovery is based on a shared problem-solving attitude and this is more likely where the patient is fully heard and fully informed.

I have been witness to recovery many, many times. In modern health care it has become possible to appreciate patients' experience, and to measure the restoration of their mental health. We need to restore our belief in the progress of mental health care. Together we can promote a response to mental suffering that overcomes the still commonplace denial and neglect of mental distress and disorder.

Now the progress of mental health needs to shift away from institutional concerns towards a focus on the personal journey of those with distress and the examination of the evidence of recovery. A new and broader vision of mental health care – with all its psychological, biological and social meanings – is emerging from the study of authentic recovery.

In the twenty-first century, the journey out of darkness into recovery has become real. We can fight the stigma of mental distress and overcome the poverty of our resources once we restore our belief in the reality of mental health recovery. Whenever we decide to take that journey together, we begin to become mentally well once again.

Everyone, regardless of diagnosis or difficulty, has a right to the expectation of recovery, which is a lasting and authentic journey of hope and human respect. As soon as we are ready to engage with that recovery, coherent and effective treatment becomes just one part of the plan for a life restored.

Caroline

Each time a new patient comes to see a psychiatrist it is a clinical experience deserving fresh attention and requiring full concentration. Clinical activity can be very intense and sometimes it is difficult to maintain this singular focus day after day. I sometimes find myself apologising to my patients for delays or interruptions that they often tolerate with true generosity.

On the day when Caroline came to my room, the distress of a previous appointment was prominent. I was relieved to hear her tell me that she was now quite well. Recognising my distraction, she spoke first, as if to reassure me by saying that she was not distressed on this occasion. She wanted to come for a routine check and to review a few things.

Then Caroline surprised me with a question. 'Why am I well? Tell me – what do you think?'

It seemed a question to which there was no clear answer, but Caroline persisted.

'I suppose you will tell me, doctor, that it is because I have taken my lithium reliably every day for the past twelve years, and that I come here to check it every four months. But somehow I think there must be more to my recovery than that.'

I asked if reconsideration of her story would help. If we did that together, might it yield a deeper understanding of Caroline's recovery?

'Yes,' she said, 'I have told you a lot about my life over the years – but it's not everything… But perhaps another time I could write it down. And I might send it to you some day. You might read it and we could talk about it if you like. Maybe I'll do that. Maybe we'll leave it for another day.'

The session ended and we both went about our day. One morning some months later, I opened my post to find a document from Caroline. There was her story, typed on the pages before me. I sat down at my desk and began to read her words.

> *I am a 58-year-old woman and I am retired from the job I have worked in for nearly twenty-five years. I am a survivor of breast cancer and it has been more than five years since my chemotherapy finished, so I see myself as being in the clear. I am not particularly courageous but I am pragmatic about things. I look forward to my retired life with my husband, Barry, my sister, Clare, and my three adult children. I hate the word 'retirement'. I prefer to call it 'choosing freedom'.*

Caroline was giving privileged access to her real self through this testimony. It is worth pondering how little any of us really knows about the life of another. Hopefully Caroline felt the value of sharing these experiences as she wrote this account, thoughtfully, quietly, somewhere in her home. Her recollection could help us both to answer her question. Why was she well?

> *These are recollections of events that occurred a long time ago. Ordinarily I work hard at putting past things away and I choose to live in the present. I don't dwell on what has gone by and, in any case, I distrust my account. It seems possible to me that these recollections may not be true memories. They are more like strong feelings which have been amplified over the years by descriptions of the events given to me by significant people in my life.*
>
> *I am told I was an anxious child and that from the start I clung tightly to my mother. In my early years it was said I would not let her out of my sight. When I was three years old, I developed*

suspected scarlet fever and I was placed for two weeks in an isolation ward. As a precaution against further infection all my clothes and toys were burned. I was the eldest of three children. My sister, Clare, was born when I was two; and my brother, Matt, when I was five. Matt was born with a severe intellectual and physical disability and so he had special needs. The family was advised to place him in an institution. In those days my parents were given very little choice. Much of their focused attention went on my brother, and his loss was a bitter event for my mother who continued to struggle with a number of further pregnancies, each ending in miscarriage, all in search of a 'perfect boy'.

Caroline's early years were significant, as they must be for each of us. It is helpful to recognise the potential of our first experiences to influence the arc of our lives, and to understand the experiences and losses that have shaped us from the start. Not every loss forms a lifelong pain and not every anxious child grows to become an anxious adult. Caroline may have been an anxious person from the start, but she experienced frightening losses early on. It remained to be seen whether she would lose out in the competition for her parents' attention and support. The experience of separation and isolation while she had scarlet fever must have been a dramatic shock. Would this be an indicator of things to come? I read on.

Our family was relatively comfortably off, as my father had a good job and he also farmed some land. For whatever reason, we were raised by a succession of mother's helpers and maids. Our parents kept an active social life and it seemed that many different people came and went from our home in Tipperary. When I was nine, and Clare was seven, we were both sent away to live with distant relatives. From then on visits from my parents were very rare but sometimes our very loving Aunt Sheila, who was my godmother, would visit us. She would bring little gifts or the occasional fruitcake and these things went some way to relieve our homesickness.

I remember on one occasion I was sent away for a two-week break in the summer holidays to be with a friend's family who had a house in Salthill in Galway. While I was out on the water a local boy set my dinghy adrift and I became inconsolably hysterical. Because of that, I was sent home in disgrace.

On the one hand Caroline had been fortunate: she had not lacked material comfort. On the other hand, there had been little real warmth or consistent affection in her early childhood. Random events and chance can have a powerful influence on the course of any of our lives. Caroline had experienced and overcome episodes of abandonment that clearly left their mark. 'For whatever reason', as Caroline had put it, there was a sense in which she was fending for herself from the very start. Nevertheless, at this stage in her life, Caroline was not blaming anyone. Her story continued.

My father had his first heart attack when I was twelve and although he appeared to have made a good recovery, he died a year later. He was only forty-eight and he had returned to work under pressure. I was sent back to boarding school with my sister a few days after his funeral, which we were not allowed to attend. At this time I was very angry with everyone in authority and most especially with my Mum. I can see now that Mum didn't handle it all very well. None of us had been at the funeral. He was carried half a mile along the road to the local church while we were bundled off to stay with local friends and I was left to explain it all to Clare. I resented the assumption that from then on I had to be an adult and to take on responsibilities for the house and most particularly responsibility for the care of my little sister.

I knew then that life had changed forever. Mum had become a farmer overnight and now Grandmother was living with us permanently. My brother, Matt, started coming home at weekends while we mostly stayed in boarding school with only one home visit each term. The care of my brother was never discussed with us and it has been a mystery to me ever since.

Reading this, the weight of tragedy in Caroline's early life was unavoidable. The early death of her father brought her childhood suddenly to an end, propelling her reluctantly into adulthood. None of this had been spoken about at the time and this distance and silence was illustrated obliquely by the lack of communication about Matt's real life in care. When it comes to recovery, timing is everything. These things were being said now because Caroline had chosen this time to share them. She went on.

After school I moved to Dublin to attend university where I took a degree in English. My happy time in college was marred by the unexpected death of Aunt Sheila, my godmother, who died in a car crash. For some reason that I cannot explain, I was not at that funeral either.

Caroline had now lost the most consistently loving figure of her childhood. To put it simply, Aunt Sheila had saved Caroline. Sheila's warm adult influence was a significant basis for the ultimate triumph that Caroline's life was to become. Recognition of the significance of positive adult influences on childhood development has been enhanced recently by the report produced by Headstrong (the national centre for youth mental health) in collaboration with the School of Psychology at University College Dublin. Their work in *My World Survey* is described as the most comprehensive survey of youth mental health ever produced in Ireland and its data highlights the positive benefit that one special adult can have on childhood development. The report states: 'One good adult is important to the mental wellbeing of young people. Over 70 per cent of young people reported that they had received high or very high levels of support from one special adult. Young people who perceived very low levels of support from a special adult when in need had significantly higher levels of depression and anxiety. The presence of one good adult is a significant indicator of how well a young person is connected, self-confident and future looking, and able to cope with problems. The absence of one good adult is linked to higher levels of distress, antisocial behaviour and an increased risk of suicidal behaviour.'

The data confirms the positive potential influence of one good adult and suggests this may be just enough to sustain the natural resilience of growing young people. In Caroline's narrative it was clear that Aunt Sheila was just such a very special person and her loss must have hit Caroline very hard. Caroline went on.

> *After graduation, I joined a volunteer programme so that I could teach overseas. My time abroad was marked with the emergence of my anxiety disorder as my first panic attacks began. I was sent to see a doctor about them, but instead of caring for me he sexually assaulted me. No one on the programme believed my story and so I returned home prematurely and told no one else of the assault for the next twenty years.*

This was a truly shocking point of Caroline's story. Who would have foreseen this revelation of sexual assault? Caroline had never spoken of this violation. She had never even hinted at it. Many people who have been victims of sexual assault never reveal their suffering and instead store their experience inside themselves until it spills over in some other context. For Caroline, the pattern of returning home in silence after unacknowledged humiliation was a recurring theme. How hard it must have been for her to trust a doctor ever again. Her generous participation in therapy over the years in her recovery seemed more and more remarkable. I read on.

On my return to Ireland I renewed my friendship with an old boyfriend, Tommy, whom I had known in my undergraduate years. We got married and moved together to Galway where he had an offer of a teaching job. At the same time, my mother remarried, but she did not tell anyone in the family and so I was not at the wedding. It was typical of my mother to go ahead with no communication. Her new husband was a stranger to all of us and the years that followed did not bring an easy resolution to our turbulent relationship.

Tommy was a good husband but our life was made very difficult by the fact that he developed a severe form of asthma and was frequently ill with many emergency hospitalisations. During the early years of our marriage we had three children: John was born first, and then Patrick, and then Jane came very prematurely at just 33 weeks. I spent six weeks prior to her birth confined to bed, lying in a single room with white walls and no view. There was so much going on at the time and there was a great deal of panic at the delivery. Sadly I had a serious manic illness after the birth and I took quite a few months to recover. I had all the features of mania and looking back it was right that I was hospitalised.

Life events came to us thick and fast. Not long after Jane was born, Tommy was made redundant. This was due in large part to his sickness record. He was never able to work again. From then on we depended entirely on my earnings, even though my job was often jeopardised by my illness. I stuck at it and eventually I was made permanent, got promoted and secured financial security for us all. I had one further manic episode but I managed to survive through most of the next twenty years even though some times were not easy.

Tommy died after a day in which he had some fleeting chest pains. He must have had a heart attack in his sleep in the night and I awoke to find him dead in the bed beside me. It was a terrible time.

Tommy's death was followed a few years later by the death of my mother, my stepfather and my brother, Matt. My mother had a long illness and died of dementia at the age of 89. Throughout this period the most constant and relevant support I had came from my sister, Clare.

It was through Clare that I met Barry, my second husband, and we have been very happy together for the past fifteen years. During my life I have been very lucky in acquiring and keeping some really good friends, although I have already lost seven to cancer. Barry in particular has played an enormous role in helping me in my recovery in recent years, visiting me when I was in hospital and keeping me connected to the outside world.

There it was. Caroline had come through and it was clear why. She has tremendous resilience. Recovery is in part about holding on. Through her Aunt Sheila and her sister, Clare, she had integrated consistent sources of love. With their support she had built a capacity for resilience that was augmented by her ability to make other supportive friendships and to keep those throughout her life. She had found a second husband who loved her and a job she could maintain. Although her youth had been full of loss and separation, her recovery had been full of communication and loving relationships.

My three children are my proudest achievement. I am relieved that they seem to be free of the anxiety and distress that characterised a lot of my life.

I am now 58 and I am well. I have three adult children who are mentally robust and I have a very satisfactory second husband. It has been twelve years since my last manic episode. That was associated with the death of my brother, Matt, and also my mother's death, which brought the ending of a very difficult relationship after a number of hard years trying to sort out her care.

Looking back, I have had a reasonable career despite my hospitalisations and I have plenty of interests in artistic activities to occupy me in my retirement. As I said, it's 'choosing freedom'. During the past decade I have purchased and refurbished our family home and this has been much more than a project. It has been part of a recovery plan that has allowed me to reoccupy my space and to find a place in it for Barry.

Caroline continued to search for answers. The answer to her recovery was complex but she still felt compelled to ask why she had become unwell in the first place.

I discovered that there is a strong history of mental illness on my father's side but I can also see now that I had a great deal of stress on me in the 1980s and 1990s. When I became the sole earner it was a time of great anxiety, with repeated hospitalisations for my mood disorder – and with Tommy's repeated hospitalisations as a result of his asthma. At one stage I had three children under the age of 5, a brother with special needs and a very ill husband.

So, why am I well now? You might say it is because of my treatment, but by my way of thinking it has also been helpful that I survived long enough to have a new and happy relationship. And my sister, Clare, has also been well and we have been able to support each other. Clare's sisterly support has helped me survive cancer and it has helped me to cope with surgery and chemotherapy. Because of my recovery I have also been able to choose freedom and to develop creative interests in things that I enjoy. Life is not a trial for me and I can look forward, not back.

There was nothing to add to her words. Caroline had answered her question. Caroline's recovery was hers – and it was a source of great joy to know that she continued to live, to learn and to love.

The Road Not Taken

Two roads diverged in a yellow wood,
And sorry I could not travel both
And be one traveler, long I stood
And looked down one as far as I could
To where it bent in the undergrowth;

Then took the other, as just as fair,
And having perhaps the better claim,
Because it was grassy and wanted wear;
Though as for that the passing there
Had worn them really about the same,

And both that morning equally lay
In leaves no step had trodden black.
Oh, I kept the first for another day!
Yet knowing how way leads on to way,
I doubted if I should ever come back.

I shall be telling this with a sigh
Somewhere ages and ages hence:
Two roads diverged in a wood, and I —
I took the one less traveled by,
And that has made all the difference.

≈

ROBERT FROST

Notes

INTRODUCTION

1   Psychiatry is a medical specialty concerned with the study, diagnosis, treatment and prevention of behavioural and mental disorders.

Psychology is the science that deals with the mind and mental processes, whether they are conscious sensations, ideas, memories or otherwise. A psychologist is a person trained as a professional in the science of psychology or a person with a degree in psychology. A clinical psychologist usually holds a doctorate degree from an accredited training programme and has at least two years of supervised experience in a clinical setting. The individual psychologist often specialises in one of the branches or fields of psychology and is identified as that type of psychologist, e.g. research psychologist or educational psychologist. They may be involved mainly in individual therapy or group therapy or any other varieties of therapeutic service provided.

2   'Countertransference' is a term taken from psychoanalysis. Broadly, it refers to the unconscious response of the therapist to the patient's personality and distress. Countertransference is considered a necessary part of the framework of recovery in classical psychoanalysis because an understanding of it contributes to the therapist's recognition of the patient's own difficulties.

The term 'countertransference' must be seen in relation to

the term 'transference'. This represents the phenomenon of
the patient's projection of his or her feelings, thoughts and
wishes onto the therapist who has come to represent an object
in the patient's own past.

EXPERIENCE
Carmel

[1]   *Bipolar mood disorder is characterised by repeated episodes in
which the patient's mood and activity levels are significantly
disturbed, this disturbance consisting on some occasions of an
elevation of mood and increased energy and activity (mania or
hypomania) and others of a lowering of mood and decreased
energy and activity (depression). Characteristically, recovery
is usually complete between episodes and the incidence in the
two sexes is more nearly equal than in other mood disorders.
As patients who suffer from repeated episodes of mania are
comparatively rare and resemble in their family history,
premorbid personality, age of onset and long-term prognosis
those who have occasional episodes of depression, such patients
are also classified as bipolar.*

   *Manic episodes usually begin abruptly and last for between
two weeks and several months. Depressions tend to last longer
though rarely last for more than one year, except in the elderly.
Episodes of both kinds often follow stressful life events or other
mental trauma but the presence of such stress is not essential
for the diagnosis. The first episode may occur at any age from
childhood to old age. The frequency of the episodes and the
pattern of remissions and relapses are both very variable,
although remissions tend to get shorter as time goes on and
depressions become commoner and longer lasting after middle
age.*

   *Although the original concept of 'manic-depressive psychosis'
also included patients who suffered only from depression, the term*

'manic-depressive disorder' is now used mainly as a synonym for bipolar disorder. Bipolar mood disorder is prevalent in the community with a rate of about 1 per cent of the population. (ICD-10)

2   Many patients use a phrase such as this to describe their episodes of depression. The particular description of melancholia as 'the black dog' is attributed to Winston Churchill. It is said that he regularly experienced bouts of melancholia.

3   Electroconvulsive therapy (ECT) is a form of physical treatment for certain mental health conditions in which an electrical current is supplied to the brain through two electrodes on the temporal areas of the skull. It can also be delivered unilaterally and this delivery may be associated with fewer side effects. The electrical current is applied through a specially constructed machine and a generalised convulsion results. ECT has been a controversial and divisive treatment that has been the focus of much attention from the anti-psychiatry movement and other critics of the medical approach to the treatment of depression. Up to 80 per cent remission is achievable in patients with depressive disorder who receive this treatment.

4   Lithium is a chemical element that is very like sodium. Whereas sodium is a salt we use to add taste to our food, lithium is found naturally in many types of mineral water. However, this is a much smaller amount than might be needed when used as a medicine. Lithium is taken in tablet form and is used to stabilise mood. It can prevent swings caused by bipolar mood disorder and it is a useful treatment in cases of mania. It can also be used to treat depression. Once commenced, lithium needs to be maintained and monitored carefully to protect against its harmful effects on the kidneys, the thyroid gland

and the heart. It may have hazardous effects when used in pregnancy. Once established, it can be used very safely when regular monitoring is put in place.

Richard

[1]   *In typical depressive episodes the individual usually suffers from lowered mood, loss of interest or enjoyment and reduced energy leading to increased fatigability and diminished activity. Marked tiredness after only slight effort is common. Other common symptoms include: reduced concentration and attention, reduced self-esteem and self-confidence, ideas of guilt and unworthiness (even in a mild type of episode), bleak and pessimistic views of the future, ideas or acts of self-harm or suicide, disturbed sleep, and diminished appetite.*

In a severe depressive episode, the sufferer usually shows considerable distress or agitation, unless retardation (slowing of the motor and cognitive functions) is a marked feature. Loss of self-esteem or feelings of uselessness or guilt are likely to be prominent, and suicide is a distinct danger in particularly severe cases. (ICD-10)

[2]   Cognitive behavioural therapy (CBT) is an active, structured and time-limited therapy that is directive and based on the belief that the way a person perceives and structures the world determines his or her feelings and behaviour. In this therapy, depression is seen as an outgrowth of a tendency to view oneself in a negative way. Treatment is aimed at altering the cognitive schema by helping the patient gather evidence for and against his or her distorted self-view. The treatment was developed by Aaron T. Beck and has its roots in earlier post-Freudian psychotherapists such as Adler, Kelly and Horney.

[3]   Selective serotonin reuptake inhibitors (SSRIs) are anti-

depressant medications that enhance the function of a brain neurotransmitter hormone known as serotonin or 5HT (5 hydroxytryptamine). The enhancement of serotonin function is associated in many with an elevation of depressed mood and a reduction in anxiety, particularly anxiety associated with obsessions and compulsions.

4   *The essential features [of panic disorder] are recurrent attacks of severe anxiety (panic) which are not restricted to any particular situation or set of circumstances and which are therefore unpredictable. As in other anxiety disorders, the dominant symptoms vary from person to person, but sudden onset of palpitations, chest pain, choking sensations, dizziness, and feelings of unreality (depersonalisation or derealisation) are common. There is also almost invariably a fear of dying, losing control, or going mad. Individual attacks usually last for minutes only, though sometimes longer... [An] individual with a panic attack often experiences a crescendo of fear and autonomic symptoms resulting in a hurried exit from wherever the panic occurs. There may be a resulting fear of going to public spaces and/or a persistent fear of having another attack.* (ICD-10)

Liam

1   'Encephalitis' refers to any inflammatory process that involves the brain. Hashimoto's encephalopathy is a rare autoimmune disorder associated with thyroid disease and with high titres of anti-thyroid antibodies. The onset tends to be insidious and is often missed by family and friends. The disorder is four times more common in women than in men. The features include recent onset of personality changes, impairment of concentration and memory difficulties, as well as headaches, muscle jerks, disorientation and confusion. Investigations reveal abnormalities of thyroid function with most people

having reduced thyroid hormone levels and also focal areas of hypo-perfusion on single photon emission brain tomography (computerised imaging of brain perfusion). Most patients respond to steroids or immune suppressant drugs so that the condition may be better described as steroid responsive acute encephalitis.

2   There is some dispute over the origin of this quotation. Nevertheless, the words are thought-provoking.

WORTH

1   'Mental distress' is a broad term for common mental problems caused by a response to stress or events. It usually represents a less severe form of suffering, usually short-term, in which the overall functioning of the person on a social, occupational or personal level continues uninterrupted.

2   'Mental disorder' is a term for less common phenomena that can occur with or without any specific stress. Severity is usually substantial and function is impacted in personal, social, occupational or other levels. Mental disorder may be defined within the diagnostic system described by the World Health Organization in ICD-10.

Alyson

1   According to ICD-10 recurrent depressive disorder *'is characterised by repeated episodes of depression without any episodes of mood elevation and over-activity that fulfil the criteria for mania'*. Episodes may be mild, moderate or severe. A moderate episode *'should have lasted a minimum of two weeks and should have been separated by several months without significant mood disturbance'*.

    'The age of onset and the severity, duration and frequency

of the episodes of depression are highly variable ... Individual episodes last between three and twelve months (median duration about six months) but recur less frequently [than bipolar mood disorder] ... Recovery is usually complete between episodes, but a minority of patients may develop persistent depression, mainly in old age ... Individual episodes of any severity are often precipitated by stressful life events; in many cultures, both individual episodes and persistent depression are twice as common in women as in men ... The risk that the patient with recurrent depressive disorder will have an episode of mania never disappears completely, however many depressive episodes he or she has experienced. If a manic episode does occur, the diagnosis should be changed to bipolar mood disorder.'

2   *Emotionally unstable personality disorder is a personality disorder in which there is a marked tendency to act impulsively without consideration of the consequences, together with affective (mood) instability. The ability to plan ahead may be minimal and outbursts of intense anger may often lead to violence or behavioural explosions; these are easily precipitated when impulsive acts are criticised or thwarted by others. F60.30 is specified as Impulsive type and its predominant characteristics are emotional instability and lack of impulse control. Outbursts of violence or threatening behaviour are common particularly in response to criticism by others. (ICD-10)*

3   *Polycystic ovarian syndrome (PCOS) is a condition in which a woman has an imbalance of female sex hormones. This may lead to menstrual cycle changes, cysts in the ovaries, trouble getting pregnant and other health changes. PCOS is linked to changes in the level of certain hormones, oestrogen and progesterone, the female hormones that help a woman's ovaries release eggs and also androgen, a male hormone found in small amounts in*

women … It is not completely understood why or how the changes in the hormone levels occur. The changes make it harder for a woman's ovaries to release fully grown (mature) eggs. Normally, one or more eggs is released during a woman's period. This is called ovulation. In PCOS, *mature eggs are not released from the ovaries. Instead, they can form very small cysts in the ovary … Some general health conditions are common in women with* PCOS *and these include diabetes mellitus, high blood pressure, high cholesterol, weight gain and obesity. Blood tests can be done to check hormone levels.* (USA National Library of Medicine)

FREEDOM
Colm

[1] *The essential feature of [obsessive-compulsive] disorder is recurrent obsessional thoughts or compulsive acts. Obsessional thoughts are ideas, images or impulses that enter the individual's mind again and again in a stereotyped form. They are almost invariably distressing (they may be violent or even obscene) or simply because they are perceived as senseless and so the sufferer often tries unsuccessfully to resist them. They are, however, recognised as the individual's own thoughts, even though they are involuntary and often repugnant.*

Compulsive acts or rituals are stereotyped behaviours that are repeated again and again. They are not inherently enjoyable, nor do they result in the completion of inherently useful tasks. The individual often views them as preventing some objectively useful event, often involving harm to or caused by him or herself. Usually, though not invariably, the individual recognises this behaviour as pointless or ineffectual and makes repeated attempts to resist it; in very long-standing cases resistance may be minimal. Autonomic anxiety symptoms (palpitations, dizziness and sweating) are often present; but distressing feelings of internal or psychic tension without obvious autonomic arousal are also common.

There is a close relationship between obsessional symptoms, particularly obsessional thoughts, and depression. Individuals with obsessive disorder often have depressive symptoms and patients with recurrent depressive disorder may develop obsessional thoughts during their episodes of depression. In either situation, increases or decreases in the severity of depressive symptoms are generally accompanied by parallel changes in the severity of obsessional symptoms.

Obsessive-compulsive disorder is equally common in men and women, and there are often prominent obsessional features in the underlying personality. Onset is usually in childhood or early adult life. The course is variable and more likely to be chronic in the absence of significant depressive symptoms. (ICD-10)

2   No medicine is completely safe. The benefits of any drug must be weighed against the extent of the hazards. Side effects are unwanted consequences of taking any treatment. They are not beneficial in themselves, but are experienced by some people and are unwelcome and potentially harmful. All medications have a potential for side effects and these are generally listed in the information attached to them when they are prescribed. For example, up to 20 per cent of people experience sexual side effects when prescribed standard antidepressants. These include a reduction in libido as well as a reduction in sexual performance.

3   Benzodiazepines (sleeping tablets) are a sedative class of medication. When they are used to induce sleep they are known as hypnotics. These medications have many other useful applications in acute critical situations in medicine, e.g. anaesthetic practice, detoxification from alcohol or acute treatment of epilepsy. Benzodiazepines are not effective antidepressants

and they are not recommended for the long-term treatment of either anxiety disorder or insomnia. When used as hypnotics, they should be withdrawn after a brief few weeks so as to avoid the development of dependency.

Brian

[1]   *The essential feature of generalised anxiety disorder is anxiety, which is generalised and persistent but not restricted to, or even strongly predominating in, any particular environmental circumstances (i.e. it is free floating). As in other anxiety disorders the dominant features are highly variable, but complaints of continuous feelings of nervousness, trembling, muscular tension, sweating, lightheadedness, palpitations, dizziness and epigastric discomfort are common. Fear that the sufferer or a relative will shortly become ill or have an accident is often expressed, together with a variety of other worries and forebodings. The disorder is more common in women and often related to chronic environmental distress. Its course is variable but it tends to be fluctuating and chronic. The sufferer must have primary symptoms of anxiety most days of the week for at least several weeks at a time, and usually for several months. The symptoms include elements of apprehension, motor tension and autonomic over-activity. The transient appearance of other symptoms, particularly depression, does not rule out generalised anxiety disorder as a main diagnosis.* (ICD-10)

MEMORY
Dorothy

[1]   *Alzheimer's disease is a primary degenerative cerebral disease of unknown cause, with characteristic neuropathological and neurochemical features. It is usually insidious in onset and develops slowly but steadily over a period of years ... There are*

characteristic changes in the brain, and a marked reduction in the population of neurons. (ICD-10)

Jack

[1] *Recurrent depressive disorder [is characterised by] a severe depressive episode ... in which the sufferer usually shows considerable distress or agitation, unless retardation is a marked feature. Loss of self-esteem or feelings of uselessness or guilt are likely to be prominent, and suicide is a distinct danger in particularly severe cases ...*

The diagnosis requires the presence of at least four of the following symptoms or signs from what is known as the somatic syndrome and these include: loss of interest or pleasure in activities that are normally enjoyable, lack of emotional reactivity to normally pleasurable surroundings or events, waking in the morning two hours or more before the usual time, depression worse in the morning, objective evidence of definite psychomotor retardation (slowing of mental processes) or agitation (remarked upon or reported by other people), marked loss of appetite, weight loss (often defined as 5 per cent or more of body weight in the past month and marked loss of libido. (ICD-10)

Margaret

[1] *Post-traumatic stress disorder arises as a delayed and/or a protracted response to a stressful event or situation of an exceptionally threatening or catastrophic nature, which is likely to cause pervasive distress in almost anyone (e.g. natural man made disaster, combat, serious accident, witnessing the violent death of others, or being the victim of torture, terrorism, rape, or other crime) ... Typical symptoms include episodes of repeated reliving of the trauma in intrusive memories (flashbacks), or dreams, occurring against the persistent sense of numbness and emotional blunting, detachment from other*

people, unresponsiveness to surroundings, anhedonia (loss of the
capacity to experience pleasure) and avoidance of activities and
situations reminiscent of the trauma. Commonly there is fear
and avoidance of cues reminiscent of the trauma. There may
be dramatic outbursts of fear, panic and aggression ... There is
usually a sustained state of autonomic hyperarousal (increased
pulse rate, sweating and rapid respiration) with hypervigilance,
an enhanced startle reaction and insomnia. Anxiety, depression
and suicidal ideation are all common. Excessive use of alcohol
and/or drugs is also seen. There is commonly a latency period
from a few weeks to a few months. The course is fluctuating but
recovery can be expected in most cases. (ICD-10)

[2]   An understanding of the role of the brain helps the
understanding of recovery. Professor Eric Kandel states
the following in *Psychiatry, Psychoanalysis and The New
Biology of Mind*: 'In so far as psychotherapy or counselling
is effective, providing long-term change in behaviour, it is
presumably effective through learning. By producing changes
in gene expression this learning alters the strength of synaptic
connections and makes structural changes which alter the
anatomical pattern of interconnections between nerve cells of
the brain.'

TRUTH
Eoin

[1]   Good sleep is essential for all health, both mental and physical,
and all mental distress is associated with disturbance of restful
sleep. Perhaps the most interesting scientist currently working
on sleep is Professor Russell Foster. His TED talk entitled 'Why
We Sleep' is a must-see for anyone interested in this area.

[2]   *A mild depressive episode is characterised by depressed mood,*

loss of interest, diminished enjoyment, and increased fatigability [and these features] are usually regarded as the most typical symptoms of depression. At least two other features from a list including the following is necessary for a reliable diagnosis: reduced concentration and attention; reduced self-esteem and self-confidence; ideas of guilt and unworthiness (even in a mild type of episode); bleak or pessimistic ideas of the future; ideas or acts of self-harm or suicide; disturbed sleep; and disturbed appetite. An individual with a mild depressive episode is usually distressed by the symptoms and has some difficulty in continuing with ordinary work and social activities, but will probably not cease to function completely. None of the symptoms should be present to an intense degree. A minimum duration of the whole episode is two weeks. (ICD-10)

3 *Morbid jealousy is a phenomenon that is more common in men than women. Many people with this unrelenting jealousy have an underlying treatable mental health disorder, and such diagnosable causes include organic brain disorders, dementias and temporal lobe disorders, bipolar mood disorders or schizophrenias. Alcohol dependence syndrome is one of the most recognized common causes. Men and women with morbid jealousy may or may not be deluded, but even without a delusional psychotic illness they can hold on to their views with such an over-valued intensity and persistence that the object of the jealous intention is unable to dispel their projection by denial or rational argument or reasoning. Sometimes the spouse can even be forced, for the sake of peace, into making a false admission and this can have disastrous consequences ...*

Alcoholic jealousy is synonymous with a cluster of psychotic phenomena [that] can occur during or immediately after psychoactive substance use, including alcohol abuse. Paranoid or persecutory ideas of reference are common and they may appear in clear consciousness. Particular care needs to be taken to avoid mistakenly making the diagnosis of schizophrenia when a diagnosis of psychoactive substance induced psychosis is actually appropriate. Many of these substance-induced states are of short duration and they can resolve completely when no further substance is taken in. This is particularly so with cases involving cocaine and amphetamines. (ICD-10)

4   *Alcohol dependence syndrome is a cluster of physiological, behavioural and cognitive phenomena in which the use of a substance takes on a much higher priority for the patient than other behaviours that once had a higher value. The diagnosis emphasises the desire and the re-establishment of the pattern even after harmful consequences are apparent. Reinstatement of harmful use even after prolonged periods of abstinence is typical.* (ICD-10)

5   The AUDIT (Alcohol Use Disorders Screening Test) can be downloaded from the WHO website: http://www.who.int/substance_abuse/publications/alcohol/en/.

BALANCE
Kathleen

1   [In mania with psychotic symptoms] *inflated self-esteem and grandiose ideas may develop into delusions and irritability, and suspiciousness into delusions of persecution. In severe cases, grandiose or religious delusions of identity or role may be prominent, and flight of ideas and pressure of speech may result in the patient becoming incomprehensible. Severe and sustained physical activity and excitement may result in aggression or violence, and neglect of eating, drinking and personal hygiene may result in dangerous states of dehydration and self-neglect.* (ICD-10)

2   There have been many theories seeking to explain the origins of bipolar mood disorder in psychological terms. We may be familiar with Freud's theories of ambivalent loss turned against the self, or Melanie Klein's concept of manic defence, in which mania is seen as protective against the pain of depression. But today very few psychiatrists believe these theories illustrate causes of bipolar disorder, even if they are helpful in descriptive terms. It is now generally accepted that the mediation of bipolar mood disorder is biological. No single physical cause is known, but the evidence from familial, hormonal, and neuropathological brain studies is compelling. While the timing of these events may have a social or psychological significance (especially in the timing of a first episode), in my experience the most significant circumstance associated with the precipitation of mania at any stage is loss of sleep.

Bipolar mood disorder is generally regarded as being present in 1 per cent of the population but, depending on the criteria used, the rates in the community may be much higher. To explain this, a number of bipolar criteria have been described. Patients who develop a cyclical mood disorder in which episodes of mania are prominent are described as Bipolar Type One. Those whose cyclical mood disorder is predominantly depressed and interrupted only by mild manias (known as hypomania) are classified as Bipolar Type Two. Still others with recurrent depression who develop mania only when exposed to antidepressant medication are sometimes called 'soft bipolars' and these are also known as Bipolar Type Three. When all three of these groups are taken together, the prevalence of bipolar mood disorder rises from 1 per cent to nearly 12 per cent of the population.

Andrew

[1]   [Mania (without psychotic symptoms) is characterised by
elevated mood that] *is out of keeping with the individual's
circumstances and may vary from carefree joviality to
almost uncontrollable excitement. Elation is accompanied by
increased energy, resulting in over activity, pressure of speech,
and a decreased need for sleep. Normal social inhibitions are
lost, attention cannot be sustained, and there is often marked
distractibility. Self-esteem is inflated, and grandiose or over-
optimistic ideas are freely expressed ...*

*Perceptual disorders may occur, such as the appreciation
of colours as especially vivid (and usually beautiful), a
preoccupation with fine details of surfaces or textures, and
subjective hyperacusis (intolerance of noise). The individual
may embark on extravagant or impractical schemes, spend
money recklessly, or become aggressive, amorous or facetious in
inappropriate circumstances. In some manic episodes the mood
is irritable and suspicious, rather than elated. The first attack
occurs commonly between the ages of 15 and 30 years, but may
occur at any age from late childhood to the seventh or eighth
decade ...*

*The episode should last for at least one week and should be
severe enough to disrupt ordinary work and social activities more
or less completely. The mood change should be accompanied
by increased energy with several of the symptoms referred
to (particularly pressure of speech, decreased need for sleep,
grandiosity and excessive optimism).* (ICD-10)

Further Reading

Barenboim, Daniel. *Everything is Connected: The Power of Music.* London: Phoenix, 2009.

Conlan, Roberta. *States of Mind.* New York: John Wiley & Sons, 1999.

Dooley, Barbara A. and Amanda Fitzgerald. *My World Survey: National Study of Youth Mental Health in Ireland.* Headstrong and School of Psychology, University College Dublin, 2012.

Ferguson, Margaret, Mary Jo Salter and Jon Stallworthy. *The Norton Anthology of Poetry.* New York: W.W. Norton & Company, 2005.

Jung, Carl Gustav. *The Undiscovered Self.* London: Routledge & Kegan Paul, 1958.

Kandel, Eric R. *Psychiatry, Psychoanalysis, and the New Biology of Mind.* American Psychiatric Press, 2005.

Knapp, Martin, David McDaid, Elias Mossialos and Graham Thornicroft. *Mental Health Policy and Practice Across Europe (European Observatory on Health Systems & Policies).* World Health Organization, 2007.

Malone, Kevin M. *Suicide in Ireland 2003–2008.* Department of Psychiatry, Psychotherapy & Mental Health Research, St Vincent's University Hospital and School of Medicine & Medical Science, University College Dublin, 2012.

National Collaborating Centre for Mental Health. *Depression: The NICE (National Institute for Health and Care Excellence) Guideline on the Treatment and Management of Depression in Adults (Updated Edition).* British Psychological Society and Royal College of Psychiatrists, 2010.

Vaillant, George E. *Triumphs of Experience.* Harvard University Press, 2012.

Wax, Ruby. *Sane New World.* London: Hodder & Stoughton, 2013.

Williams, Mark and Danny Penman. *Mindfulness: A Practical Guide to Finding Peace in a Frantic World.* London: Piatkus, 2011.

World Health Organization. *International Classification of Diseases (ICD): Tenth Revision.* World Health Organization, 1990.